CASES IN

Microscopic Haematology

CASES IN Microscopic Haematology

Gillian Rozenberg

CHURCHILL LIVINGSTONE
ELSEVIER

Sydney Edinburgh London New York Philadelphia St Louis Toronto

Churchill Livingstone
is an imprint of Elsevier

Elsevier Australia. ACN 001 002 357
(a division of Reed International Books Australia Pty Ltd)
Tower 1, 475 Victoria Avenue, Chatswood, NSW 2067

National Library of Australia Cataloguing-in-Publication Data

---

Rozenberg, Gillian.

Cases in microscopic haematology / Gillian Rozenberg.

9780729540926 (pbk.)

Hematology – Case studies.
Blood – Diseases – Case studies.

616.15

Publisher: Melinda McEvoy
Developmental Editor: Rebecca Cornell
Publishing Services Manager: Helena Klijn
Project Coordinator: Natalie Hamad
Edited by Elaine Cochrane
Proofread by Forsyth Publishing Services
Picture research by Copper Leife
Cover and internal design by Lisa Petroff
Typeset by Midland Typesetters
Printed by CTPS

Contents

Acknowledgements

There are a number of people to whom I am indebted for their assistance with the production of this book.

I would like to thank Professor Robert Lindeman, the Director of the Department of Haematology at the Prince of Wales Hospital, for allowing me access to the blood films and bone marrows in our laboratory, Virginia Bentink for her expertise in producing all 106 images, and Narelle Woodland, Senior Lecturer and Coordinator of Haematology at the University of Technology, Sydney, for her support during the writing of this book.

Reviewers

Anne-Marie Christensen, BAppSc(Med Lab Sci), BSc(Hons), MAppSc(Med Sci)
MAIMS, AACB, MIBMS
Discipline of Medical Sciences, Faculty of Science & Technology, Queensland University of Technology

Angus Fraser, FIBMS, CSci
Singapore Polytechnic
Institute of Biomedical Science (IBMS), UK

Chris Kendrick, GradDipSci, MSc(Dis)
NZ Registered Medical Laboratory Scientist, Senior Lecturer in Haematology & Transfusion Science
Massey University

Gweneth F MacDonald, BAppSci (Med Lab), DipEd (TAFE)
AAIMLS
Royal Melbourne Institute of Technology (RMIT), Melbourne

Valerie Ng, PhD MD
Alameda County Medical Center
University of California San Francisco
Professor Emeritus, Department of Laboratory Medicine, School of Medicine, UCSF; Chair, Laboratory Medicine & Pathology, Alameda County Medical Center; Director, ACMC Clinical Laboratory

E P Theakston, MBChB, FRCPA
Labplus
Auckland District Health Board

Craig Williams, BAppSci (Med Lab)
MAIMS
Sullivan Nicolaides Pathology

1 Examination of the Blood Film

A well made, well stained blood film is the key to a clear, accurate interpretation of the findings under the microscope.

PREPARATION OF THE BLOOD FILM

Blood is collected into the anticoagulant ethylenediamine tetra acetic acid (EDTA) dipotassium salt at a concentration of 1.50 ± 0.25 mg/mL. The ratio of blood to EDTA is critical as excess EDTA results in shrinkage and degeneration of the cells, especially the red cells.

The quality of the blood film is directly related to the quality of the materials used to produce it. The glass slides must be of a high quality. Pre-cleaned slides with frosted ends are preferable and, for safety, the slides should have bevelled edges. The spreader used to produce the blood film should also be of a high quality with bevelled edges.

- Dry the blood film in front of a cold-air fan placed in the safety cabinet immediately after it has been spread.
- Fix the blood film in AR grade methanol.
- Stain in Wright's stain or another Romanowsky stain.
- Coverslip the blood film using a good quality mountant.

Examine the blood film systematically.

- On **low power** (×10 objective) check the tail for platelet clumping as well as the number and distribution of the white cells.
- Check for the presence of rouleaux and correlate the degree of rouleaux with the ESR result.
- On **high power** (×40 objective) perform a white cell differential.
- Estimate and correlate the platelet count with the result issued by the blood cell analyser.
- Examine the red cells as to their size, shape and colour.
- On **oil immersion** (×100 objective) examine for the presence of malarial parasites on the thick film only (the thin film is examined using the ×40 objective).
- Check for red cell inclusions when indicated.
- Perform manual reticulocyte counts.

ARTIFACTUAL CHANGES SEEN ON THE BLOOD FILM

Red cell artifact

- Old blood: storing blood in EDTA for more than 6 hours will lead to progressive red cell crenation.
- Incorrect ratio of blood to EDTA is usually due to difficulty in collection of the specimen. Excess EDTA induces shrinkage of red cells.
- Moisture in the methanol produces rings in the red cells, giving a false impression of hypochromasia.
- Slow drying of the blood film allows moisture from the atmosphere to be absorbed onto the surface of the red cells, increasing the surface area unevenly and inducing the appearance of 'pseudo' target cells.
- Action of heat on red cells gives rise to the presence of spherocytes as well as red cell fragments, which in turn will lead to a false high platelet count.

White cell artifact

- Old blood: when blood is stored in EDTA for more than 24 hours vacuoles will be seen in the cytoplasm of the neutrophils and monocytes. The nuclei of the neutrophils will become degenerate. The lobes will separate and become pyknotic, a process known as apoptosis.
- Crush artifact: white cells may be crushed during spreading of the blood film, especially the lymphocytes of lymphoproliferative disorders. Such crushed cells are known as smudge cells or smear cells. This artifact may be minimised by the addition of albumin (1 drop of 30% albumin to 9 drops of blood) and then spreading the blood film.

Platelet artifact

- Difficult collection: incorrect venepuncture technique can induce platelet aggregation or clumping. Always examine the film, especially the tail of the film, when the platelet count is unexpectedly reduced.
- Platelet satellitism is usually due to the presence of immunoglobulins, potentiated by EDTA, which induce platelet adherence to the neutrophil membrane. The presence of platelet satellitism will lead to a falsely reduced platelet count.
- Stain quality: stain precipitate on the film, incorrect stain time, incorrect ratio of stain to buffer, and incorrect pH of the buffer can all contribute to poor stain quality.

RED CELLS

Red cells should be examined in an area where they are just touching. Keep away from the tail as well as the thicker part of the film, especially if rouleaux is present.

How to Use this Book

Cases in Microscopic Haematology is a compilation of 80 haematology cases representing red cell, white cell, platelet and malaria disorders and neoplasms and encompassing all age groups. A valuable resource for students, scientists and medical registrars in haematology in its own right, this collection of case studies will be most useful when used in conjunction with the author's *Microscopic Haematology* 3rd edition (Churchill Livingstone, Sydney, 2011).

Chapter 1 describes how to prepare a good quality blood film. The film is examined systematically, avoiding mention of any red cell, white cell or platelet artifact that may be present and ensuring that the parameters issued by the analyser correlate with those seen under the microscope. A blood film comment is performed using the standard nomenclature, grading the changes according to the number of cells seen on the blood film, either slight, moderate or marked.

A description is provided of the artifactual changes that may occur in red cells, white cells and platelets, followed by a section on red cell nomenclature that contrasts the appearance of red cells on a stained blood film with their appearance under the electron microscope. White cell and platelet maturation are also described, referring to the images as they appear in *Microscopic Haematology* 3rd edition.

The case studies have been divided into chapters of red cell, white cell, platelet and malaria cases. Many of these cases will have a differential diagnosis.

Consider case study 20, a 25-year-old Asian female who is 4 weeks pregnant. The analyser data and the blood film indicate that this patient has a microcytic hypochromic anaemia. From this evidence, the reader should be able to arrive at the differential diagnosis of iron deficiency, thalassaemia, or a combination of both. The reader is then asked which further tests would be requested by the clinician in order to make an actual outcome or definitive diagnosis.

Case study 38 is that of a 64-year-old male with lassitude, anaemia and splenomegaly. The analyser data identifies a very high white cell count. The reader should recognise that the white cell count and differential are pathognomonic of a particular myeloproliferative neoplasm; however, further tests – a bone marrow and cytogenetics – will be requested by the clinician in order to make a definitive diagnosis.

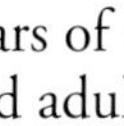 indicates a paediatric case. The reference ranges for neonates, infants and children differ from those in adults. This difference continues until twelve years of age when, haematologically, children are considered comparable to adults and adult reference ranges can be applied. Many clinical conditions that occur in the paediatric patient are not seen in adults; conversely, many clinical conditions that occur in adults are infrequent in the paediatric patient.

The differential diagnosis, further tests, and the actual outcome or diagnosis of each case study will be found in the Answers section, with additional explanation where appropriate.

Acknowledgements

There are a number of people to whom I am indebted for their assistance with the production of this book.

I would like to thank Professor Robert Lindeman, the Director of the Department of Haematology at the Prince of Wales Hospital, for allowing me access to the blood films and bone marrows in our laboratory, Virginia Bentink for her expertise in producing all 106 images, and Narelle Woodland, Senior Lecturer and Coordinator of Haematology at the University of Technology, Sydney, for her support during the writing of this book.

ARTIFACTUAL CHANGES SEEN ON THE BLOOD FILM

Red cell artifact

- Old blood: storing blood in EDTA for more than 6 hours will lead to progressive red cell crenation.
- Incorrect ratio of blood to EDTA is usually due to difficulty in collection of the specimen. Excess EDTA induces shrinkage of red cells.
- Moisture in the methanol produces rings in the red cells, giving a false impression of hypochromasia.
- Slow drying of the blood film allows moisture from the atmosphere to be absorbed onto the surface of the red cells, increasing the surface area unevenly and inducing the appearance of 'pseudo' target cells.
- Action of heat on red cells gives rise to the presence of spherocytes as well as red cell fragments, which in turn will lead to a false high platelet count.

White cell artifact

- Old blood: when blood is stored in EDTA for more than 24 hours vacuoles will be seen in the cytoplasm of the neutrophils and monocytes. The nuclei of the neutrophils will become degenerate. The lobes will separate and become pyknotic, a process known as apoptosis.
- Crush artifact: white cells may be crushed during spreading of the blood film, especially the lymphocytes of lymphoproliferative disorders. Such crushed cells are known as smudge cells or smear cells. This artifact may be minimised by the addition of albumin (1 drop of 30% albumin to 9 drops of blood) and then spreading the blood film.

Platelet artifact

- Difficult collection: incorrect venepuncture technique can induce platelet aggregation or clumping. Always examine the film, especially the tail of the film, when the platelet count is unexpectedly reduced.
- Platelet satellitism is usually due to the presence of immunoglobulins, potentiated by EDTA, which induce platelet adherence to the neutrophil membrane. The presence of platelet satellitism will lead to a falsely reduced platelet count.
- Stain quality: stain precipitate on the film, incorrect stain time, incorrect ratio of stain to buffer, and incorrect pH of the buffer can all contribute to poor stain quality.

RED CELLS

Red cells should be examined in an area where they are just touching. Keep away from the tail as well as the thicker part of the film, especially if rouleaux is present.

Classification

- Size (anisocytosis)
  The red cell distribution width (RDW) is the index of anisocytosis.
  Larger cells are known as macrocytes and smaller cells as microcytes.
- Shape (poikilocytosis)
  Poikilocytes are red cells of abnormal shape that are produced as a result of abnormal erythropoiesis, pathological conditions, or inherited disorders.
- Colour
  Normochromasia, hypochromasia, hyperchromasia and polychromasia.

Red cell distribution width

The RDW is an index of anisocytosis or variation in red cell size. Anisocytosis is reported as a degree in the variation of red cell size. It will be either slight (+), moderate (++) or marked (+++). The presence of reticulocytes, which are larger than mature red cells, should be excluded when assessing the degree of anisocytosis.

Anisocytosis is a significant parameter in many red cell disorders and may be used as a guide in the differential diagnosis of certain anaemias.

- RDW-CV (RR <14.5) / RDW-SD (RR <48).
- The RDW is increased in iron deficiency and decreased in children between the ages of 6 months and 5 years (who may also be iron deficient).
- The RDW is decreased in thalassaemia trait and increased in thalassaemia intermedia and thalassaemia major. It is increased in myelodysplastic syndromes.
- A moderate degree of anisocytosis should be qualified by the presence of microcytes as well as macrocytes.

Shape

The morphological abnormalities seen in red cells on a well spread, well stained blood film offer a key to the interpretation of a particular pathological condition. Conversely, certain pathological conditions may be attributed to the presence of certain red cell shapes on the blood film.

With this in mind, the morphologist must be ever mindful of the standard nomenclature used to describe red cell shapes. The ability to recognise 'true' red cell shapes as opposed to those produced artifactually in vitro is vital to an accurate film report. The degree used to describe the number of red cell shapes may also have a clinical significance. In general, the morphologist should not comment on red cell shapes occurring 'occasionally' on the blood film. A slight, moderate or marked number of red cell shapes are suggestive of a pathological condition. The use of the term 'occasional' may confuse the clinical diagnosis.

The use of the term 'poikilocyte' to describe variation in red cell shape should be discouraged. Every red cell that is not a biconcave disc or discocyte is a poikilocyte. If there are red cell changes on the film, report those individual changes. By reporting this way the diagnosis will be clear to both the morphologist and the clinician.

Nomenclature

Normal red cells (discós = disc / discocyte)

Normal red cells are biconcave discs or discocytes. They have a mean diameter of 7 µm and are approximately the size of a small lymphocyte nucleus.

The red cell membrane is very elastic and deformable, readily able to reassume its discoidal shape after cessation of a deforming force.

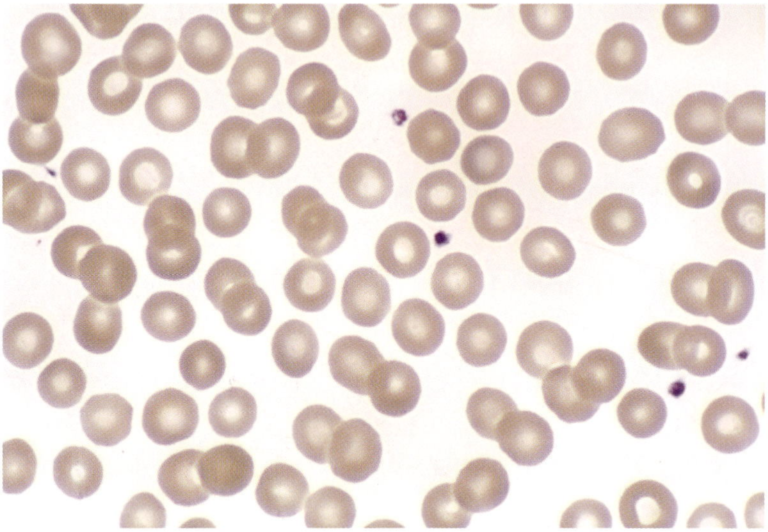

Normal red cells

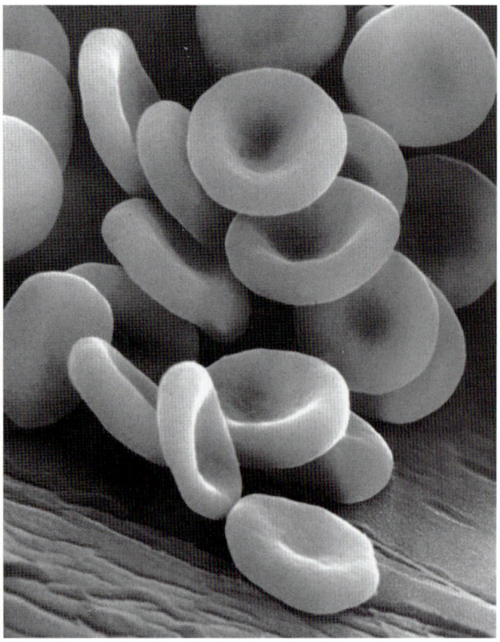

Normal red cells

Microcytes (micrós = small)

Microcytes are red cells with a diminished diameter, less than 6 µm, and diminished thickness. The haemoglobin concentration of microcytes is reduced and often concentrated in a peripheral ring, while the centre is pale. This pale centre may be so increased in size that the cell resembles a leptocyte or a thin, flattened red cell. Microcytes are a characteristic feature of iron deficiency and/or thalassaemia.

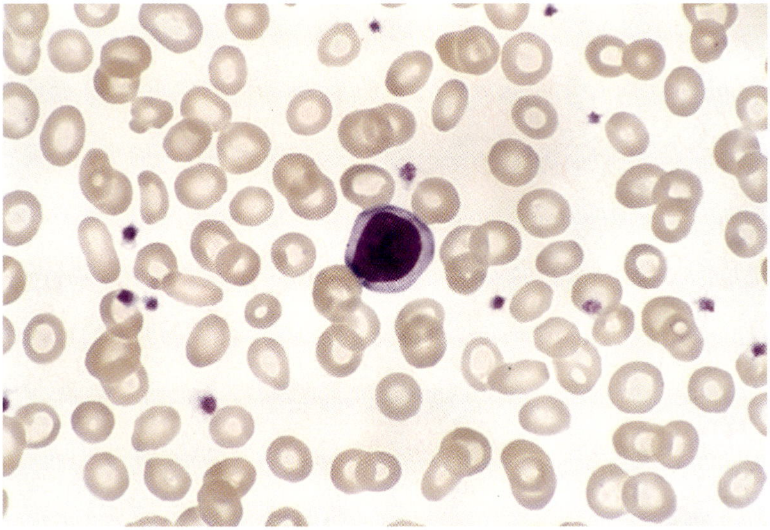

Microcytes

Macrocytes (macrós = large)

Macrocytes are red cells with an increased diameter, more than 8 µm. They maintain a normal discoid shape and have a well defined central depression. Macrocytes are a characteristic feature of alcoholism and liver disease.

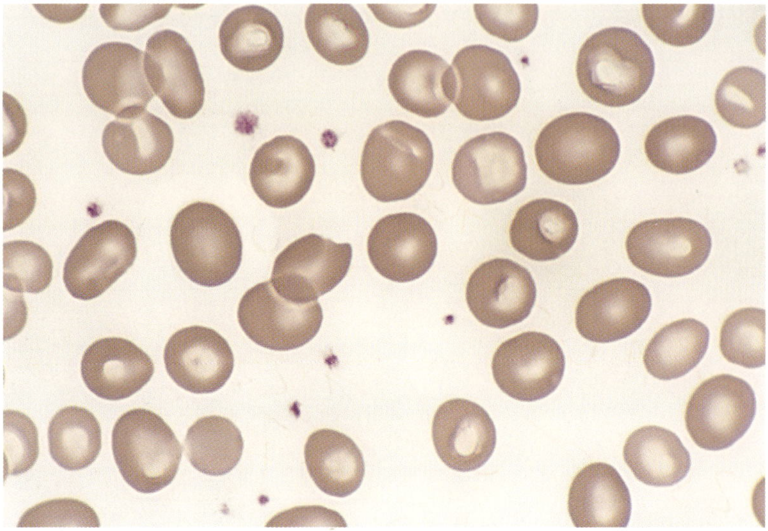

Macrocytes

Oval macrocytes (macrós = large)

Oval macrocytes are giant sized red cells with a diameter of more than 9 µm. They are a characteristic feature of megaloblastic anaemia (mégas = giant).

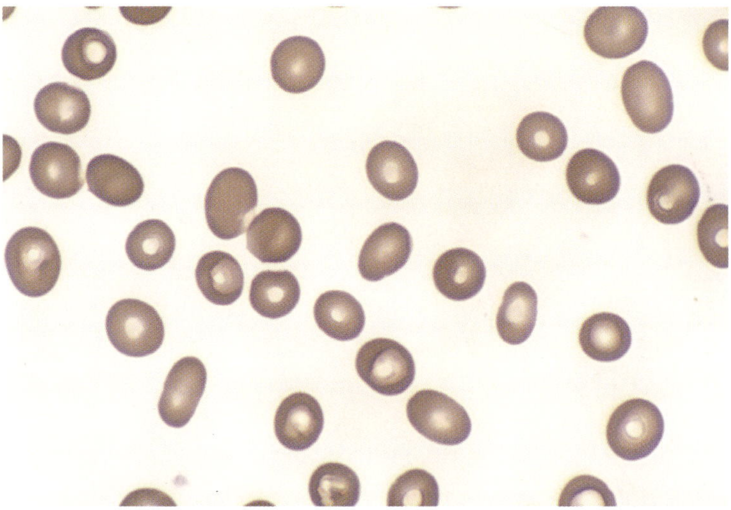

Oval macrocytes

Target cells (kódon = bell / codocyte)

Target cells are bell-shaped, thin-walled cells that have an increased surface area compared to volume. This is the result of red cell membrane expansion by the accumulation of lecithin and cholesterol from free exchange with plasma lipids. The term 'target' describes the appearance of these cells when dried on a glass slide. They have a characteristic distribution of haemoglobin in the centre of the cell as well as around the periphery, with the two regions separated by a pale ring. Target cells are associated with liver disease, thalassaemia, hyposplenism, and some abnormal haemoglobins.

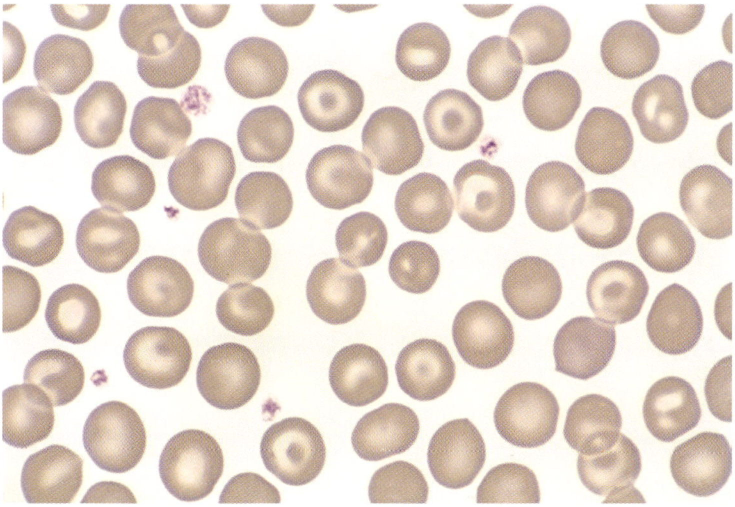

Target cells

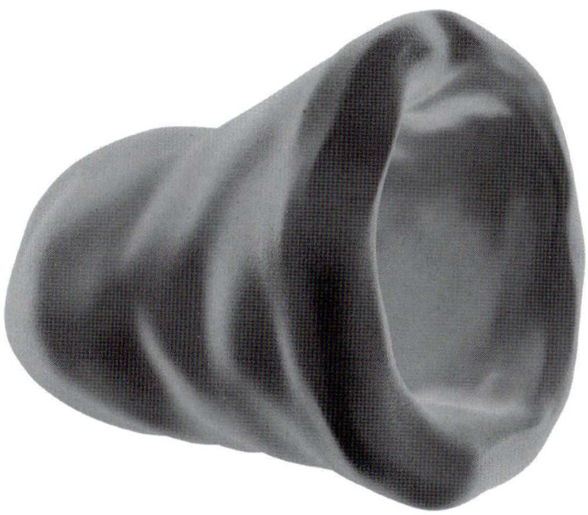

Target cell

Elliptocytes (elleiptikós = elliptic)

Elliptocytes are oval biconcave discs that vary in shape from slightly oval to cylindrical. They have both a quantitative and qualitative abnormality in spectrin and protein 4.1, two major proteins comprising the membrane skeleton.

Approximately 5% of red cells seen in normal blood films are elliptocytes, but in hereditary elliptocytosis between 30% and 100% of red cells are elliptocytes.

Elliptocytes are also a feature of iron deficiency anaemia, but without the spectrin or protein 4.1 abnormality.

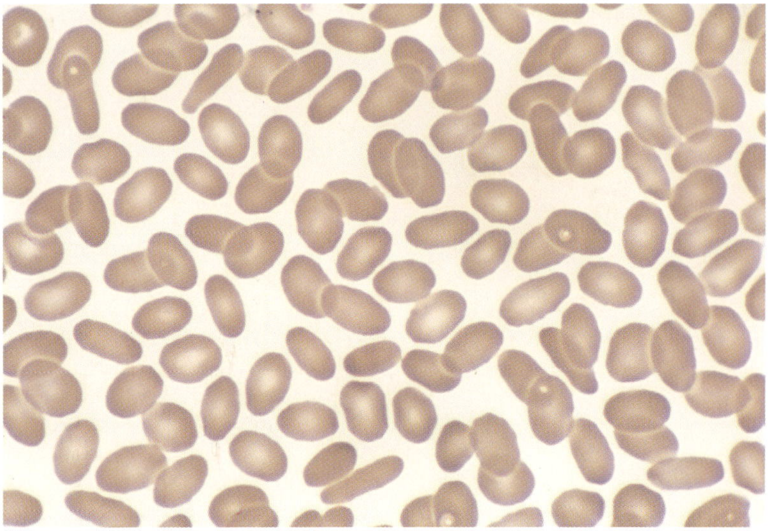

Elliptocytes

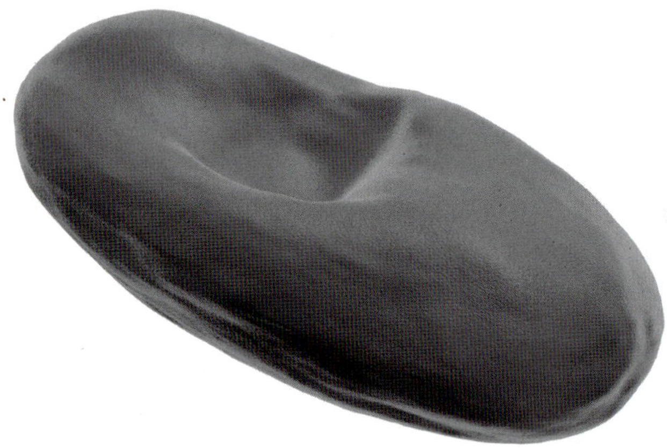

Elliptocyte

Stomatocytes (stóma = mouth)

Stomatocytes are bowl-shaped red cells that exhibit a slit-like area of central pallor. They are associated with alcoholism and also a feature of hereditary stomatocytosis and Southeast Asian ovalocytosis. The membrane defect is different in each of these conditions. Stomatocytes may also occur in vitro as an artifact of improper physicochemical conditions.

In hereditary stomatocytosis there is a deficiency of protein 7.2b or stomatin in the red cell membrane. This deficiency leads to an influx of Na^+ into the red cell and a loss of K^+ exiting the red cell. Hence the red cells swell and are transformed from discocytes to bowl forms. They have a high mean cell volume (MCV), usually about 130 fL.

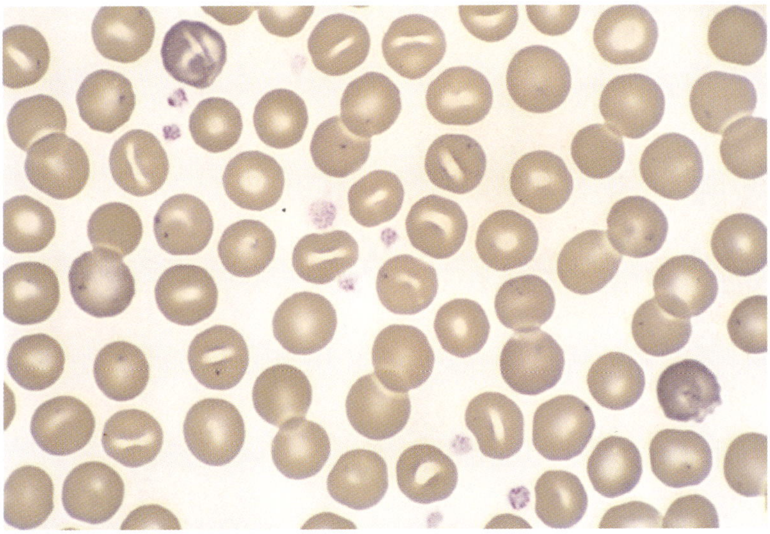

Stomatocytes of hereditary stomatocytosis

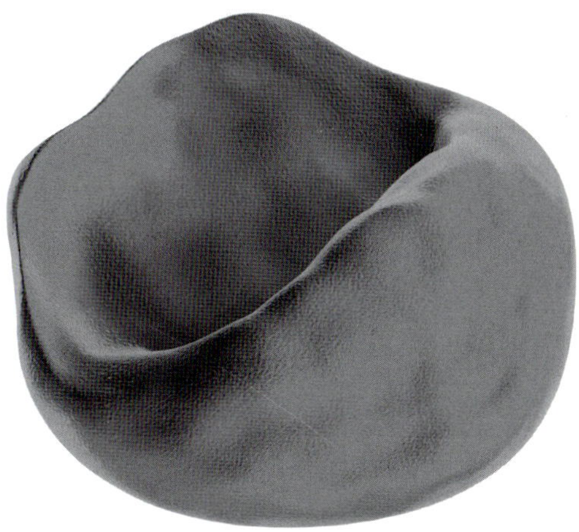

Stomatocyte of hereditary stomatocytosis

In Southeast Asian ovalocytosis, there is increased ankyrin binding and decreased protein 3 mobility, leading to the production of rigid red cells, oval in shape, often with double transverse slits. They have a normal MCV.

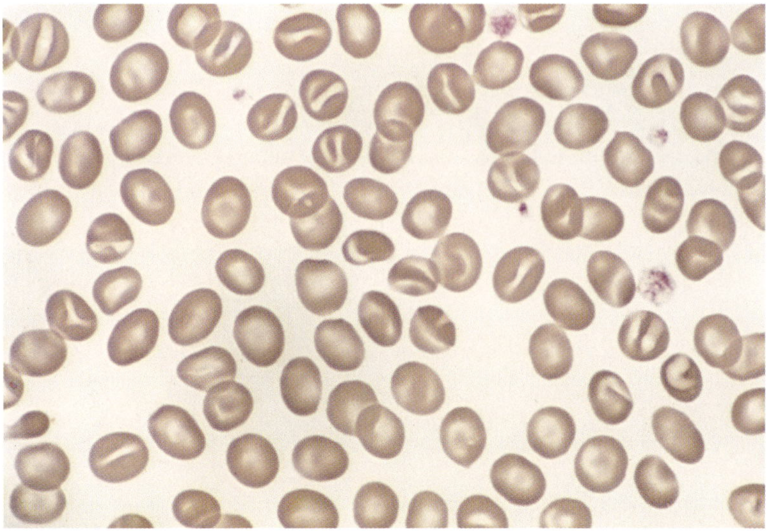

Stomatocytes of Southeast Asian ovalocytosis

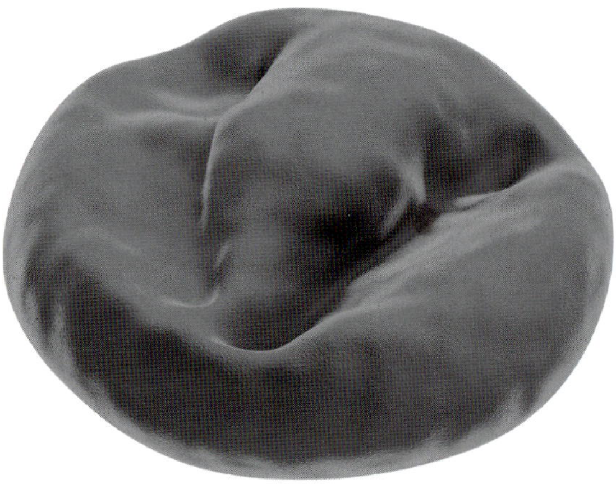

Stomatocyte of Southeast Asian ovalocytosis

Spherocytes (sfáira = sphere)

Spherocytes are red cells that are almost spherical in shape; they are no longer a biconcave disc. They appear as slightly smaller, hyperchromic red cells with little or no area of central pallor. The MCV of spherocytes is within the normal range.

Spherocytes are a characteristic feature of hereditary spherocytosis and autoimmune haemolytic anaemia. The spherocytes of hereditary spherocytosis are attributable to an intracorpuscular red cell membrane defect. Deficiency of spectrin, ankyrin or band 3 protein leads to the uncoupling of the skeletal lipid bilayer, resulting in membrane loss in the form of microvesicles.

The spherocytes of autoimmune haemolytic anaemia are the end result of the coating of red cells with immunoglobulin, namely IgG and/or complement proteins.

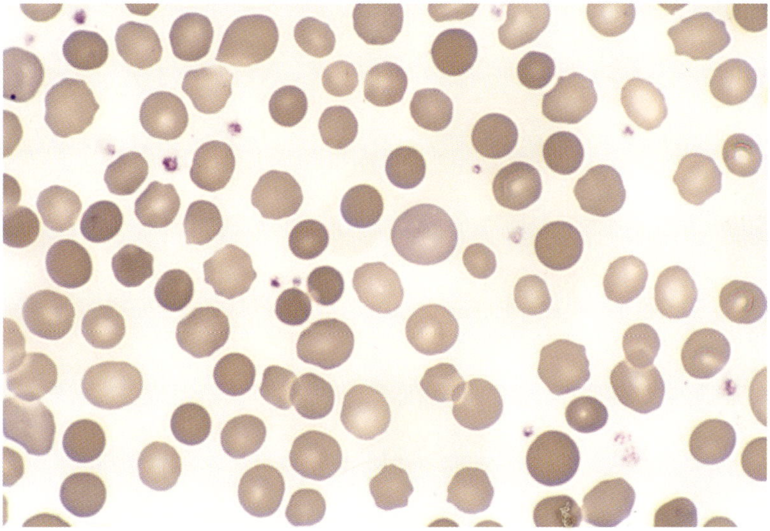

Spherocytes

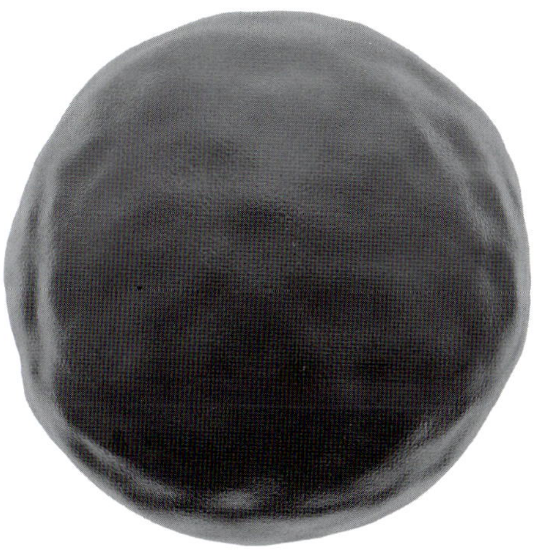

Spherocyte

Sickle cell (drepánon = sickle / drepanocyte)

Sickle cells are biconcave discs that, upon deoxygenation, change shape to become crescent or sickle-shaped. They have an abnormal haemoglobin, HbS, which is produced by the replacement of glutamic acid with valine at the sixth position on the β chain.

Sickle cells are deformed by the precipitation of polymerised HbS. They appear as sickle or crescent-shaped red cells on the blood film.

As well as being a characteristic feature of sickle cell disease, sickle cells are also a feature of double-heterozygote disorders that include HbS.

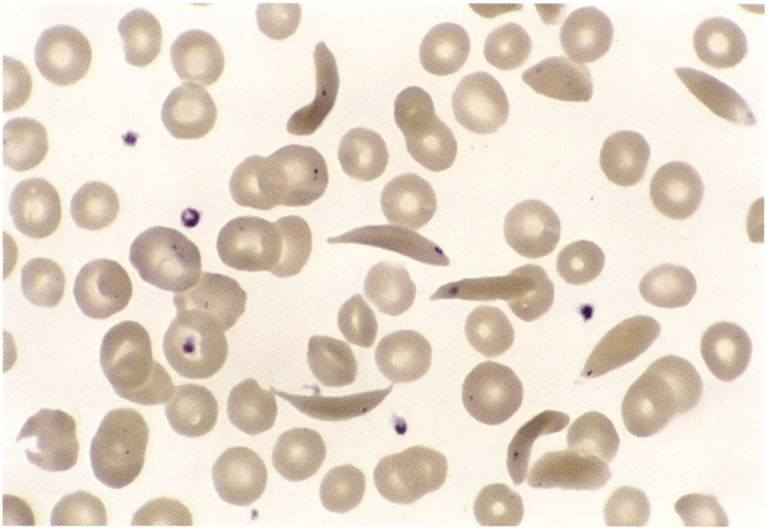

Sickle cells

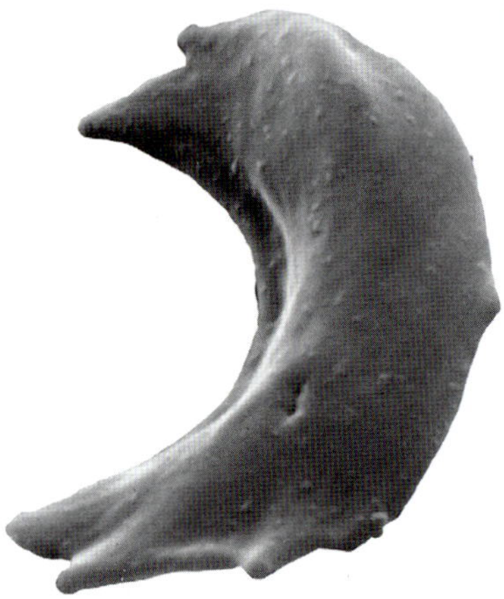

Sickle cell

Teardrops (dákryon = tear / dacryocyte)

Teardrop-shaped red cells are characterised by a single elongated or pointed extremity. They are a characteristic feature of leucoerythroblastic disorders such as myelofibrosis and metastatic carcinoma.

Teardrops are also present in thalassaemia and megaloblastic anaemia.

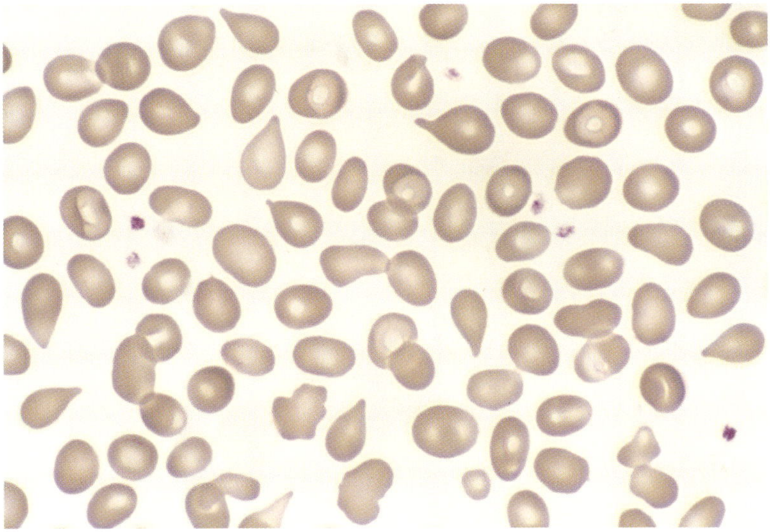

Teardrops

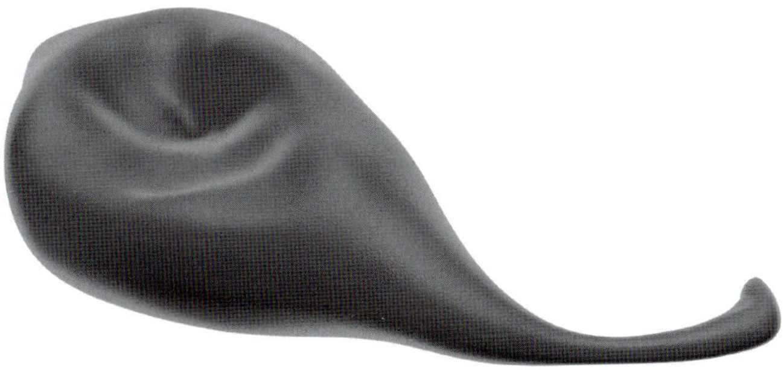

Teardrop

Acanthocytes (ákanta = spine)

Acanthocytes are round, hyperchromic red cells with several fine, spine-like projections spaced unevenly over their entire surface. They are a characteristic feature of hyposplenism and splenectomy, abetalipoproteinaemia, and the McLeod phenotype.

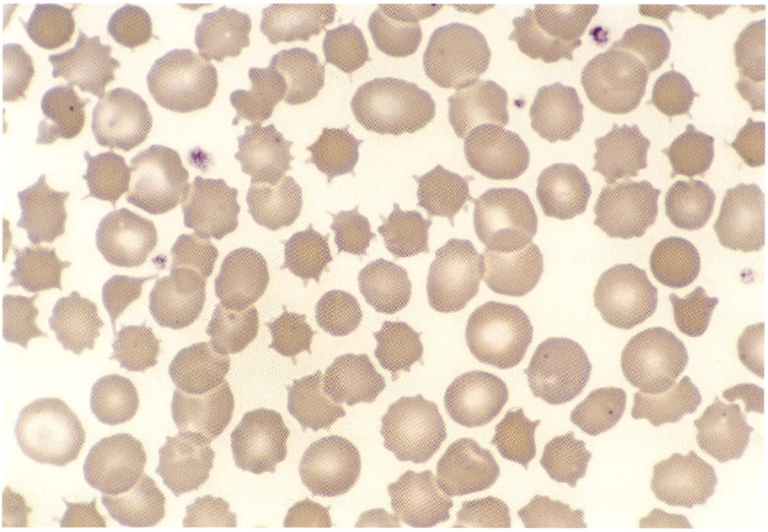

Acanthocytes

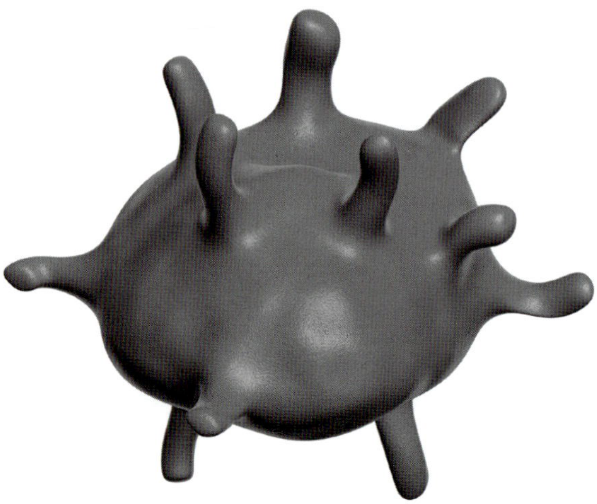

Acanthocyte

Bite / blister cells (dángo = bite / dangocyte)

Bite cells are formed when Heinz bodies (the product of oxidant stress on the haemoglobin molecule), together with some red cell content, are removed from red cells as they pass through the spleen. A blister-like structure forms when the red cell membrane repairs around the bite, hence the term 'blister cell'.

Bite and blister cells are a characteristic feature of oxidant haemolysis seen in subjects with normal and reduced levels of glucose 6 phosphate dehydrogenase (G6PD). They may also appear after the administration of oxidant drugs, for example dapsone, salazopyrin, bactrim, and some of the antimalarial drugs.

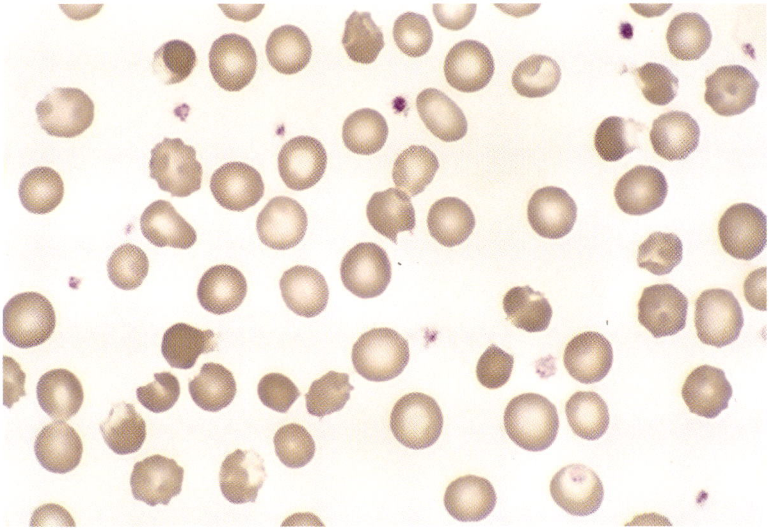

Bite cells and blister cells

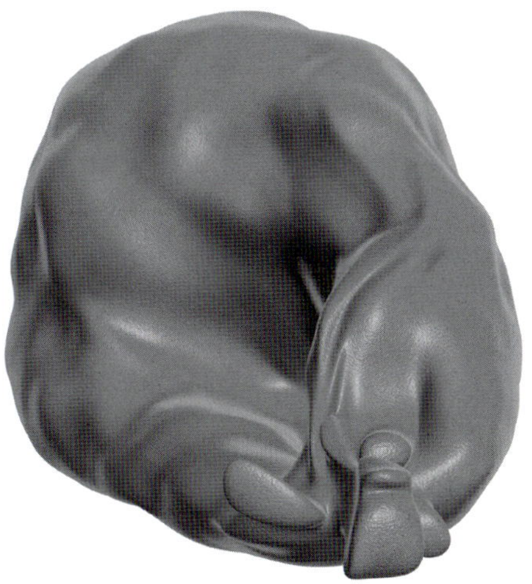

Blister cell

Schistocytes (skiss = rip)

Schistocytes are sharp, pointed fragmented red cells produced by a microangiopathic process. Red cells are fractured or ripped as they pass across strands of fibrin in damaged vessels, for example in haemolytic uraemic syndrome (HUS), or as they pass across a damaged or prosthetic heart valve.

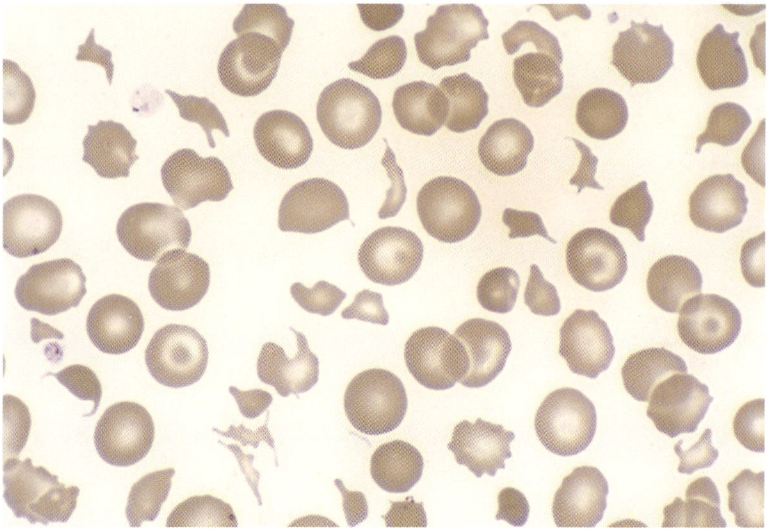

Schistocytes

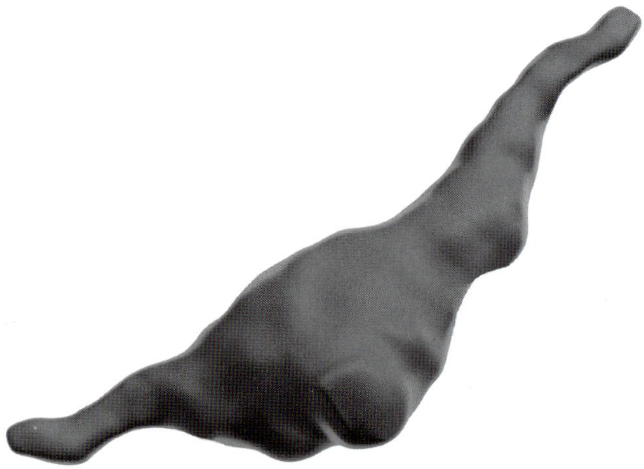

Schistocyte

Crenated cells (échin = sea urchin / echinocyte stage 1)

Crenated cells are red cells with irregularly placed projections on their surface. They are invariably present as an artifact that develops if blood is allowed to stand for a prolonged period of time at 20°C before the films are made. Crenated cells present in freshly made blood films are a feature of renal disease. They are also present in dehydration resulting from severe gastroenteritis, especially in young children.

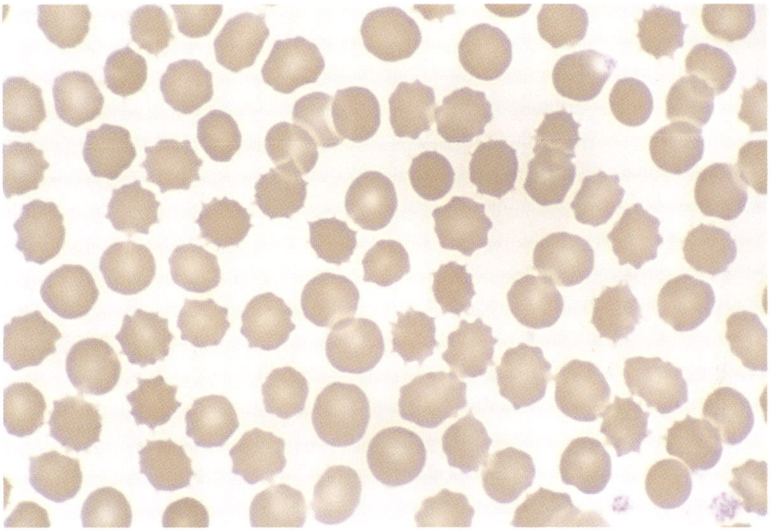

Crenated cells

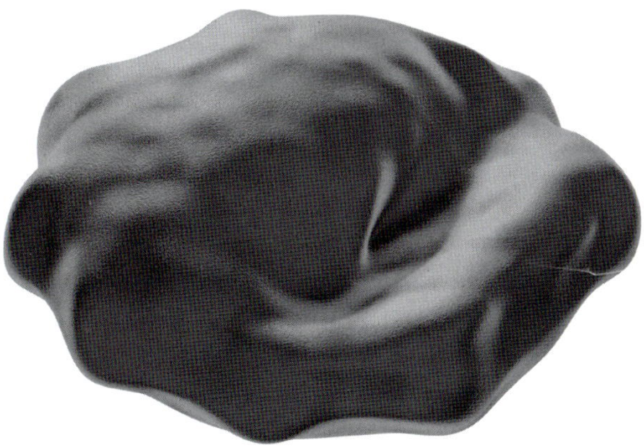

Crenated cell

Burr cells (échin = sea urchin / echinocyte stage 2)

Burr cells are red cells with varying numbers of spines occurring at irregular intervals on the red cell membrane. They are produced as a result of damaged glomeruli in severe glomerulonephritis and in acute renal failure.

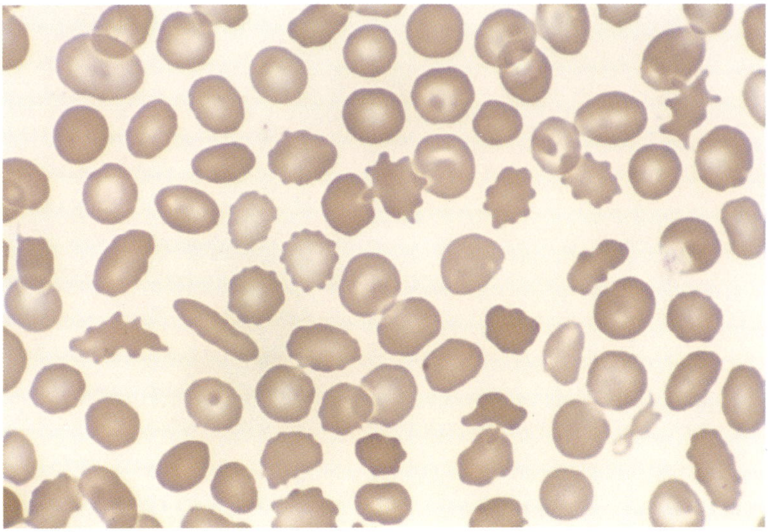

Burr cells

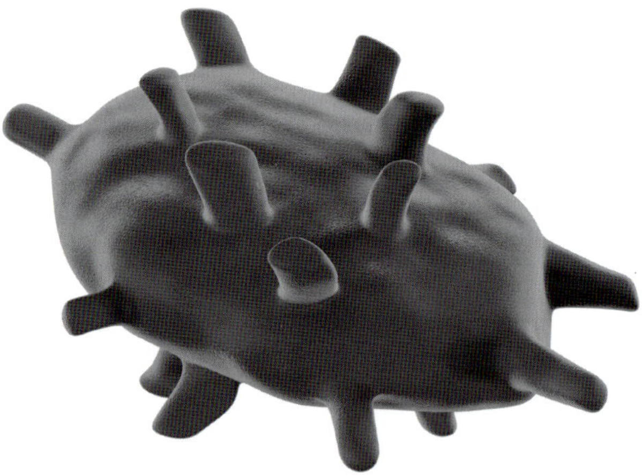

Burr cell

Spur cells (échin = sea urchin / echinocyte stage 3)

Spur cells are spiculated red cells, with equally spaced short spines over the entire surface of the red cell. They appear as three-dimensional on the blood film.

Spur cells are produced in two stages. First, excess cholesterol produced by the diseased liver increases the surface area of the red cell membrane, resulting in a red cell with a scalloped or undulating periphery. Second, these scalloped cells are converted to spur cells by a process of splenic conditioning. Over a period of a few days, the membrane lipids as well as the increased surface area are lost, and the cell becomes rigid, assuming the appearance of a spur cell.

Spur cells are characteristic of fulminant hepatocellular disease. This haematological condition is commonly referred to as spur cell anaemia.

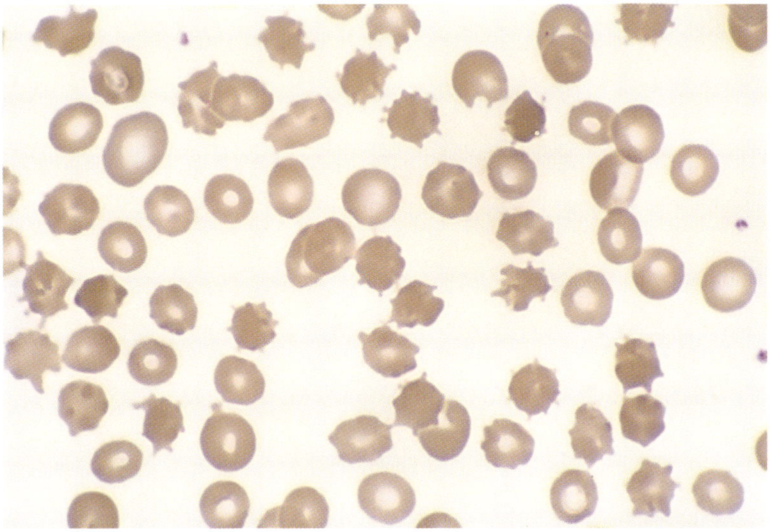

Spur cells

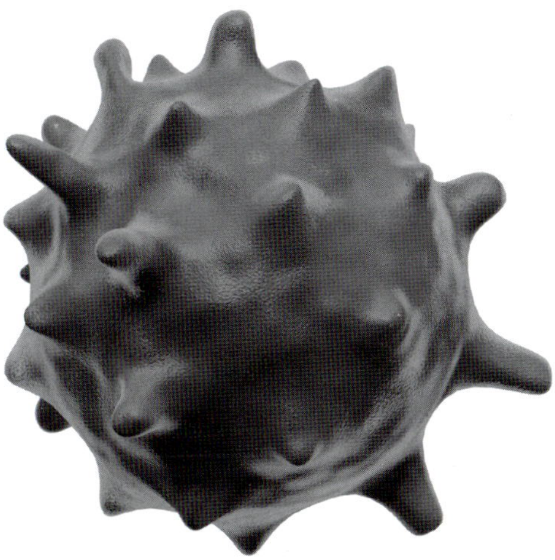

Spur cell

WHITE CELLS

Myeloid cells

Myeloblast

The myeloblast varies from 15 to 20 μm in diameter and has a large round nucleus that occupies about 80% of the cell. The chromatin is arranged in fine strands, giving an evenly stained reticular appearance with approximately one to three nucleoli. The cytoplasm is very basophilic and agranular. Refer to Figure B1-1 in *Microscopic Haematology* 3rd edn.

Promyelocyte

The promyelocyte is the next stage in the maturation process. It is approximately the same size as the myeloblast. The nucleus still contains nucleoli, but the chromatin strands are coarser and hence stain less evenly. The cytoplasm is still basophilic but now contains azurophilic or primary granules. Refer to Figure B1-2 in *Microscopic Haematology* 3rd edn.

Myelocyte

The myelocyte may be up to 25 μm in diameter. The nucleus is round and the chromatin strands are thicker and stain more deeply than in the promyelocyte. There are no nucleoli present. The nuclear to cytoplasmic (N/C) ratio is decreased. Primary granules may be seen in the early myelocyte while the late or more developed myelocyte contains specific or secondary granules. Refer to Figures B1-3 to B1-4 in *Microscopic Haematology* 3rd edn.

Metamyelocyte

The metamyelocyte, which is between 10 and 18 μm in diameter, is characterised by an indented nucleus resembling the shape of a broad bean. The chromatin strands are thicker and stain more deeply than in the myelocyte, and the cytoplasm contains many fine specific granules. Refer to Figure B1-5 in *Microscopic Haematology* 3rd edn.

Band form

The band form, 10–15 μm in diameter, is smaller than the metamyelocyte. It has a deeply indented U-shaped nucleus composed of coarsely clumped chromatin. The cytoplasm is pink and contains many specific granules. Refer to Figure B1-6 in *Microscopic Haematology* 3rd edn.

Neutrophil

The neutrophil is approximately 12–14 μm in diameter. The nucleus is lobulated, having three or four lobes connected by thin strands of chromatin. The cytoplasm is pink and contains specific granules. Refer to Figure B1-7 in *Microscopic Haematology* 3rd edn.

Eosinophil

The mature eosinophil is a round cell, 12–17 µm in diameter. It is characterised by the presence of large round granules with an affinity for acid dyes such as eosin. The nucleus has two or three lobes. Eosinophils are attracted to sites of antigen–antibody interaction in tissues, especially in cases of foreign protein sensitisation such as allergic disorders and parasitic infections. Refer to Figure B1-8 in *Microscopic Haematology* 3rd edn.

Basophil

The basophil is a round cell approximately 10–14 µm in diameter; its nucleus is bilobed. The granules are large and bluish-black in colour and are present in the cytoplasm as well as overlying and partly obscuring the nucleus. Refer to Figure B1-9 in *Microscopic Haematology* 3rd edn.

Monocytes

Monoblast

The monoblast varies in diameter from 14 to 18 µm. It has a round to oval nucleus occupying about 80% of the cell. One or two nucleoli are present. The cytoplasm is basophilic and lacks granules. Refer to Figure B2-1 in *Microscopic Haematology* 3rd edn.

Promonocyte

The promonocyte varies in diameter from 14 to 18 µm. The nucleus is indented and often contains a nucleolus. The cytoplasm is blue-grey and may contain a few fine azurophilic granules. Refer to Figure B2-2 in *Microscopic Haematology* 3rd edn.

Monocyte

The monocyte varies in diameter from 12 to 18 µm. The nucleus is folded and lobulated, with two or more lobes. The cytoplasm is grey-blue with numerous fine azurophilic granules. Vacuolation is a characteristic feature of the mature monocyte. Refer to Figure B2-4 in *Microscopic Haematology* 3rd edn.

Lymphocytes

Lymphoblast

The lymphoblast varies from 10 to 20 µm in diameter. It has a round nucleus that occupies about 80% of the cell. The chromatin is fine and contains one or two nucleoli. The cytoplasm is basophilic and agranular. Refer to Figure B4-1 in *Microscopic Haematology* 3rd edn.

Prolymphocyte

The prolymphocyte varies in diameter from 10 to 18 µm. The nucleus is round, the chromatin denser and the cytoplasm more abundant than in the lymphoblast. One prominent nucleolus is present within the nucleus. Refer to Figure B4-2 in *Microscopic Haematology* 3rd edn.

Lymphocyte (small)

The small lymphocyte varies in diameter from 9 to 12 µm. The nucleus is round, with coarse clumped chromatin. The cytoplasm is scanty, sky-blue in colour, and agranular. Refer to Figure B4-3 in *Microscopic Haematology* 3rd edn.

Lymphocyte (large)

The large lymphocyte varies in diameter from 12 to 16 µm. The nucleus is round, with coarse clumped chromatin. The cytoplasm is abundant and sky-blue in colour, and often contains a few fine azurophilic granules. Refer to Figure B4-4 in *Microscopic Haematology* 3rd edn.

Reactive lymphocyte

The reactive lymphocyte has a round to irregularly shaped nucleus with abundant flowing cytoplasm that characteristically has a dark-staining periphery. Refer to Figure B4-5 in *Microscopic Haematology* 3rd edn.

Plasma cells

Plasmablast

The plasmablast varies from 16 to 18 µm in diameter and has a round nucleus occupying about 80% of the cell. The chromatin is fine and contains one to three nucleoli. The nucleus is usually eccentrically placed within intensely basophilic cytoplasm; a perinuclear halo, representing the Golgi apparatus, may be present. Refer to Figure B5-3 in *Microscopic Haematology* 3rd edn.

Proplasma cell

The proplasma cell varies from 15 to 25 µm in diameter and has a round eccentrically placed nucleus containing one to three nucleoli. The cytoplasm is intensely basophilic, with a perinuclear halo. Refer to Figure B5-4 in *Microscopic Haematology* 3rd edn.

Plasma cell

The plasma cell varies from 8 to 20 µm in diameter. It has a round eccentrically placed nucleus with dense chromatin pattern. The cytoplasm is basophilic with a perinuclear halo. Refer to Figure B5-6 in *Microscopic Haematology* 3rd edn.

PLATELETS

Refer to Part B3 in *Microscopic Haematology* 3rd edn.

MALARIAL PARASITES

Refer to Part D1 in *Microscopic Haematology* 3rd edn.

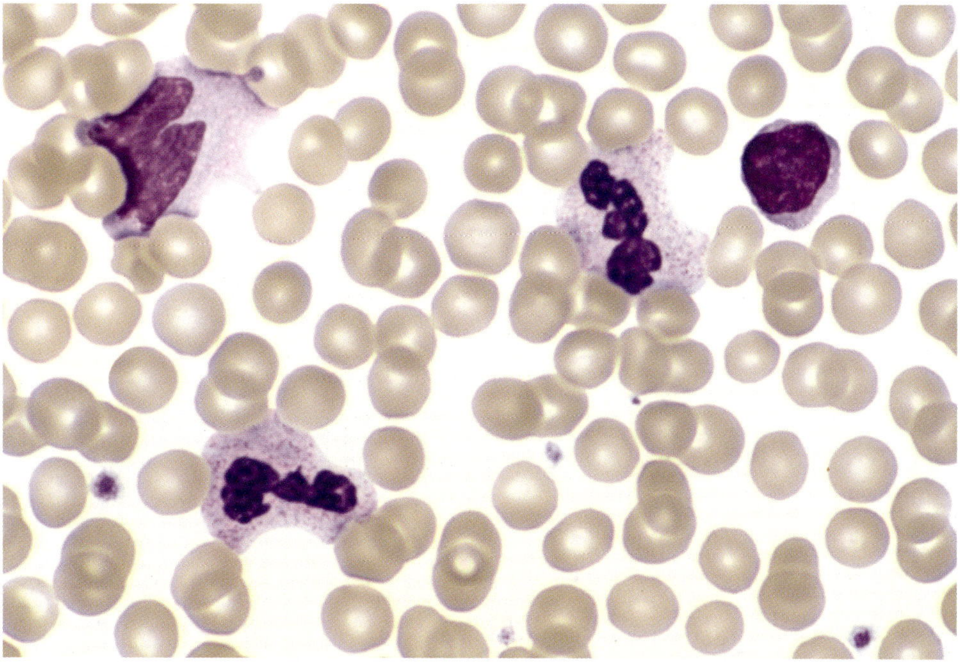

Blood film comments	
Red cell comments	Red cells normal in number and morphology
White cell comments	White cells normal in number and morphology
Platelet comments	Platelets normal in number and morphology

Question 1. What is the differential diagnosis?

Based on the differential diagnosis, the following tests should be requested
Not applicable.

Question 2. Are further tests indicated as part of your final report? If so, which tests?

CASE STUDY 2

Case history

A 48-year-old female with a history of menorrhagia.

Analyser data				
Parameters	**Test Results**		**Reference Range**	
RBC	4.32	× 10^{12}/L	3.80–5.80	× 10^{12}/L
Hb	60	g/L	115–165	g/L
HCT	0.180		0.37–0.47	
MCV	58.3	fL	80–100	fL
MCH	13.9	pg	26.5–33.0	pg
MCHC	238	g/L	310–360	g/L
RDW-SD	53.7	fL	38.0–48.0	fL
RDW-CV	16.5	%	12.0–14.5	%
RETIC CT	0.9	%	0.2–2.0	%
RETIC ABS	38.9	× 10^9/L	20–80	× 10^9/L
WBC	9.4	× 10^9/L	3.5–11.0	× 10^9/L
Plat	438	× 10^9/L	150–400	× 10^9/L

Differential						
Parameters	**Test Results**				**Reference Range**	
Neutrophil	72.2	%	6.8	× 10^9/L	1.7–7.0	× 10^9/L
Lymphocyte	20.9	%	2.0	× 10^9/L	1.5–4.0	× 10^9/L
Monocyte	4.7	%	0.4	× 10^9/L	0.1–0.8	× 10^9/L
Eosinophil	2.0	%	0.19	× 10^9/L	0.04–0.44	× 10^9/L
Basophil	0.2	%	0.02	× 10^9/L	0.00–0.20	× 10^9/L

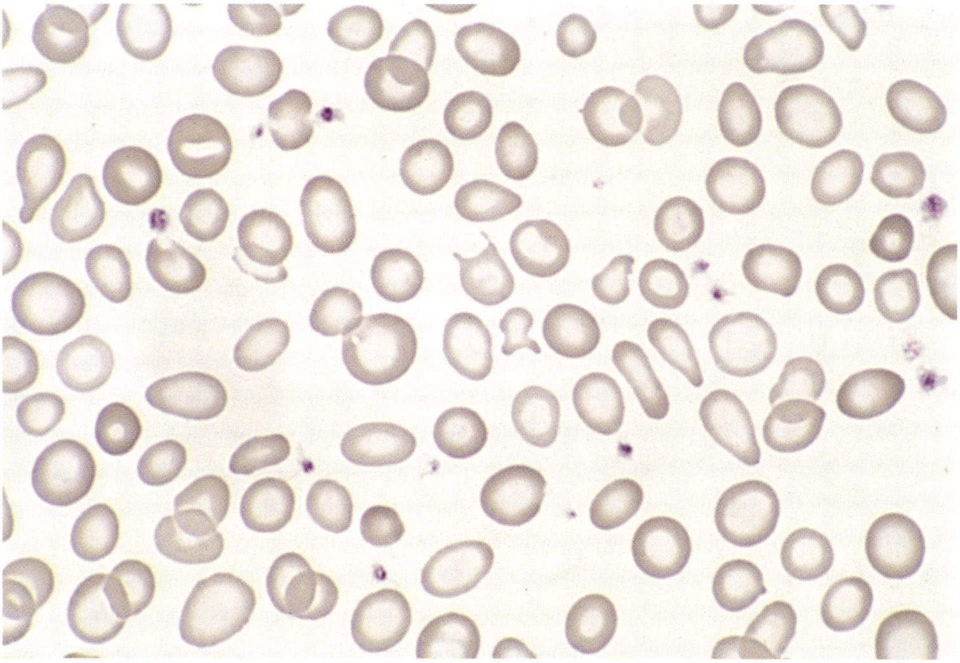

Blood film comments	
Red cell comments	Slight anisocytosis Marked microcytes Marked hypochromasia Slight elliptocytes Slight pencil cells
White cell comments	White cells normal in number and morphology
Platelet comments	Thrombocytosis

Question 1. What is the differential diagnosis?

Based on the differential diagnosis, the following tests should be requested				
Iron studies				
Iron	1.7	µmol/L	RR (8.1–32.6)	µmol/L
Transferrin	4.2	g/L	RR (1.8–3.3)	g/L
Iron saturation	1.6	%	RR (20–52)	%
Ferritin	2.0	µg/L	RR (20–300)	µg/L

Question 2. Are further tests indicated as part of your final report? If so, which tests?

CASE STUDY 3

Case history

A 48-year-old female with a history of menorrhagia post completion of a course of oral iron.

Analyser data				
Parameters	**Test Results**		**Reference Range**	
RBC	4.91	$\times 10^{12}/L$	3.80–5.80	$\times 10^{12}/L$
Hb	102	g/L	115–165	g/L
HCT	0.304		0.37–0.47	
MCV	73.2	fL	80–100	fL
MCH	25.7	pg	26.5–33.0	pg
MCHC	323	g/L	310–360	g/L
RDW-SD	58.4	fL	38.0–48.0	fL
RDW-CV	18.1	%	12.0–14.5	%
RETIC CT				
RETIC ABS				
WBC	8.8	$\times 10^9/L$	3.5–11.0	$\times 10^9/L$
Plat	450	$\times 10^9/L$	150–400	$\times 10^9/L$

Differential						
Parameters	**Test Results**				**Reference Range**	
Neutrophil	72.9	%	6.4	$\times 10^9/L$	1.7–7.0	$\times 10^9/L$
Lymphocyte	18.6	%	1.6	$\times 10^9/L$	1.5–4.0	$\times 10^9/L$
Monocyte	6.2	%	0.5	$\times 10^9/L$	0.1–0.8	$\times 10^9/L$
Eosinophil	2.1	%	0.18	$\times 10^9/L$	0.04–0.44	$\times 10^9/L$
Basophil	0.2	%	0.02	$\times 10^9/L$	0.00–0.20	$\times 10^9/L$

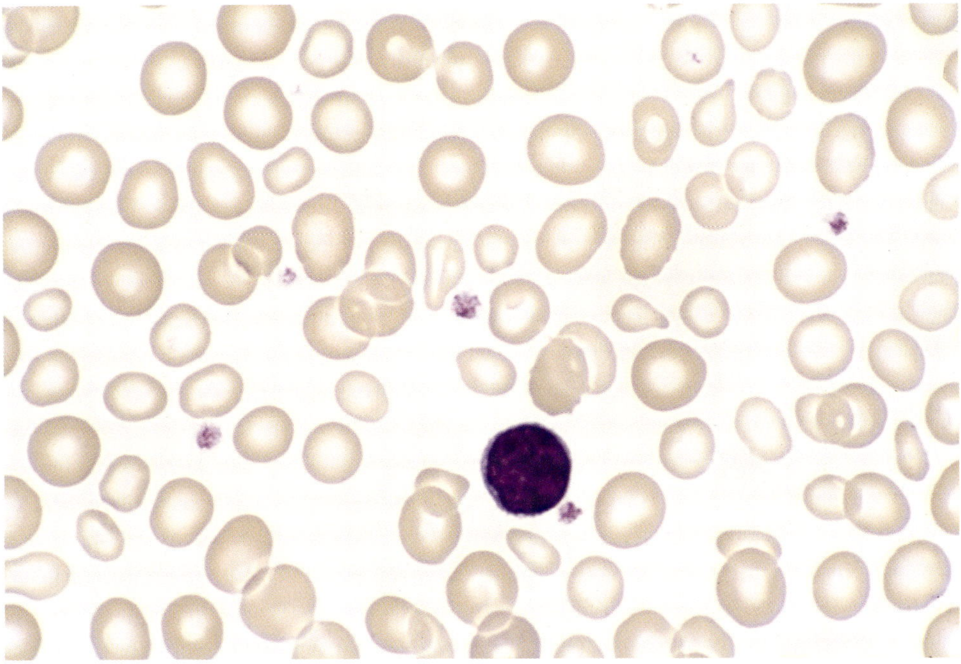

Blood film comments	
Red cell comments	Moderate anisocytosis Slight microcytes Slight hypochromasia Slight elliptocytes Slight pencil cells Dimorphic film
White cell comments	White cells normal in number and morphology
Platelet comments	Thrombocytosis

Question 1. What is the differential diagnosis?

Based on the differential diagnosis, the following tests should be requested
Not applicable.

Question 2. Are further tests indicated as part of your final report? If so, which tests?

CASE STUDY 4

Case history

A 75-year-old male presents with shortness of breath.

Analyser data				
Parameters	**Test Results**		**Reference Range**	
RBC	1.26	$\times 10^{12}$/L	4.50–6.50	$\times 10^{12}$/L
Hb	49	g/L	130–180	g/L
HCT	0.159		0.40–0.54	
MCV	126.2	fL	80–100	fL
MCH	38.9	pg	26.5–33.0	pg
MCHC	308	g/L	310–360	g/L
RDW-SD	86.4	fL	38.0–48.0	fL
RDW-CV	50.7	%	12.0–14.5	%
RETIC CT	0.1	%	0.2–2.0	%
RETIC ABS	1.26	$\times 10^9$/L	20–80	$\times 10^9$/L
WBC	3.2	$\times 10^9$/L	3.5–11.0	$\times 10^9$/L
Plat	113	$\times 10^9$/L	150–400	$\times 10^9$/L

Differential						
Parameters	**Test Results**				**Reference Range**	
Neutrophil	60	%	1.9	$\times 10^9$/L	1.1–6.0	$\times 10^9$/L
Lymphocyte	35	%	1.1	$\times 10^9$/L	2.7–8.9	$\times 10^9$/L
Monocyte	4	%	0.1	$\times 10^9$/L	0.2–1.1	$\times 10^9$/L
Eosinophil	1	%	0.03	$\times 10^9$/L	0.0–0.6	$\times 10^9$/L
Basophil	0	%	0.00	$\times 10^9$/L	0.00–0.10	$\times 10^9$/L

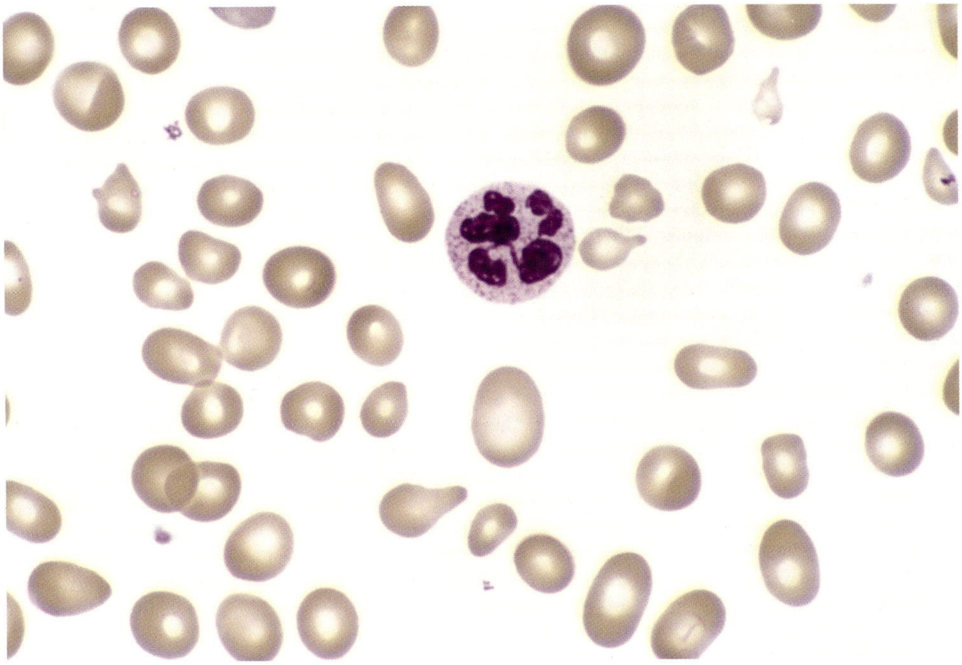

Blood film comments	
Red cell comments	Moderate anisocytosis Marked oval macrocytes Slight microcytes Slight teardrop poikilocytes
White cell comments	Hypersegmented neutrophils Lymphopenia
Platelet comments	Thrombocytopenia

Question 1. What is the differential diagnosis?

Based on the differential diagnosis, the following tests should be requested				
Serum B_{12}	56	pmol/L	RR (109–646)	pmol/L
Serum folate	>45.3	nmol/L	RR (6.5–40.5)	nmol/L
Red cell folate	>2000	nmol/L	RR (539–1685)	nmol/L

Question 2. Are further tests indicated as part of your final report? If so, which tests?

CASE STUDY 5

Case history

A 10-month-old child presents with fever; he is pale and lethargic.

Analyser data

Parameters	Test Results		Reference Range	
RBC	1.25	$\times 10^{12}$/L	3.88–5.13	$\times 10^{12}$/L
Hb	40	g/L	104–132	g/L
HCT	0.124		0.30–0.38	
MCV	99.2	fL	70–83	fL
MCH	32.0	pg	23.1–29.4	pg
MCHC	323	g/L	310–360	g/L
RDW-SD	82.1	fL	34.8–44.6	fL
RDW-CV	53.5	%	12.3–17.0	%
RETIC CT	0.1	%	0.2–2.0	%
RETIC ABS	1.25	$\times 10^{9}$/L	20–80	$\times 10^{9}$/L
WBC	5.9	$\times 10^{9}$/L	5.4–13.6	$\times 10^{9}$/L
Plat	42	$\times 10^{9}$/L	205–553	$\times 10^{9}$/L

Differential

Parameters	Test Results				Reference Range	
Neutrophil	20.5	%	1.2	$\times 10^{9}$/L	1.1–6.0	$\times 10^{9}$/L
Lymphocyte	70.3	%	4.1	$\times 10^{9}$/L	2.7–8.9	$\times 10^{9}$/L
Monocyte	7.0	%	0.4	$\times 10^{9}$/L	0.2–1.1	$\times 10^{9}$/L
Eosinophil	0.8	%	0.05	$\times 10^{9}$/L	0.0–0.6	$\times 10^{9}$/L
Basophil	1.4	%	0.08	$\times 10^{9}$/L	0.00–0.20	$\times 10^{9}$/L

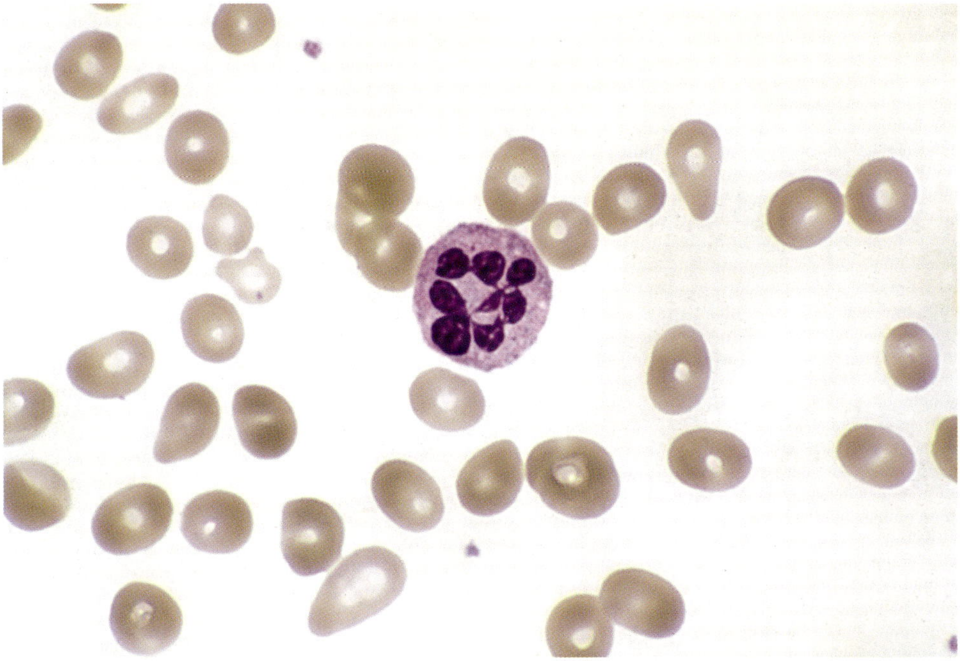

Blood film comments	
Red cell comments	Moderate anisocytosis Moderate oval macrocytes Slight teardrop poikilocytes
White cell comments	Hypersegmented neutrophils
Platelet comments	Thrombocytopenia

Question 1. What is the differential diagnosis?

Based on the differential diagnosis, the following tests should be requested				
Serum B_{12}	100	pmol/L	RR (97–394)	pmol/L
Serum folate	2.1	nmol/L	RR (5.5–33.3)	nmol/L

Question 2. Are further tests indicated as part of your final report? If so, which tests?

CASE STUDY 6

Case history
A 45-year-old male found collapsed on the floor.

Analyser data				
Parameters	**Test Results**		**Reference Range**	
RBC	4.41	$\times 10^{12}$/L	4.50–6.50	$\times 10^{12}$/L
Hb	151	g/L	130–180	g/L
HCT	0.453		0.40–0.54	
MCV	99.8	fL	80–100	fL
MCH	34.2	pg	26.5–33.0	pg
MCHC	343	g/L	310–360	g/L
RDW-SD	52.1	fL	38.0–48.0	fL
RDW-CV	15.7	%	12.0–14.5	%
RETIC CT				
RETIC ABS				
WBC	11.1	$\times 10^9$/L	3.5–11.0	$\times 10^9$/L
Plat	71	$\times 10^9$/L	150–400	$\times 10^9$/L

Differential						
Parameters	**Test Results**				**Reference Range**	
Neutrophil	82.9	%	9.2	$\times 10^9$/L	1.7–7.0	$\times 10^9$/L
Lymphocyte	7.1	%	0.8	$\times 10^9$/L	1.5–4.0	$\times 10^9$/L
Monocyte	7.2	%	0.8	$\times 10^9$/L	0.1–0.8	$\times 10^9$/L
Eosinophil	2.5	%	0.28	$\times 10^9$/L	0.04–0.44	$\times 10^9$/L
Basophil	0.3	%	0.03	$\times 10^9$/L	0.00–0.20	$\times 10^9$/L

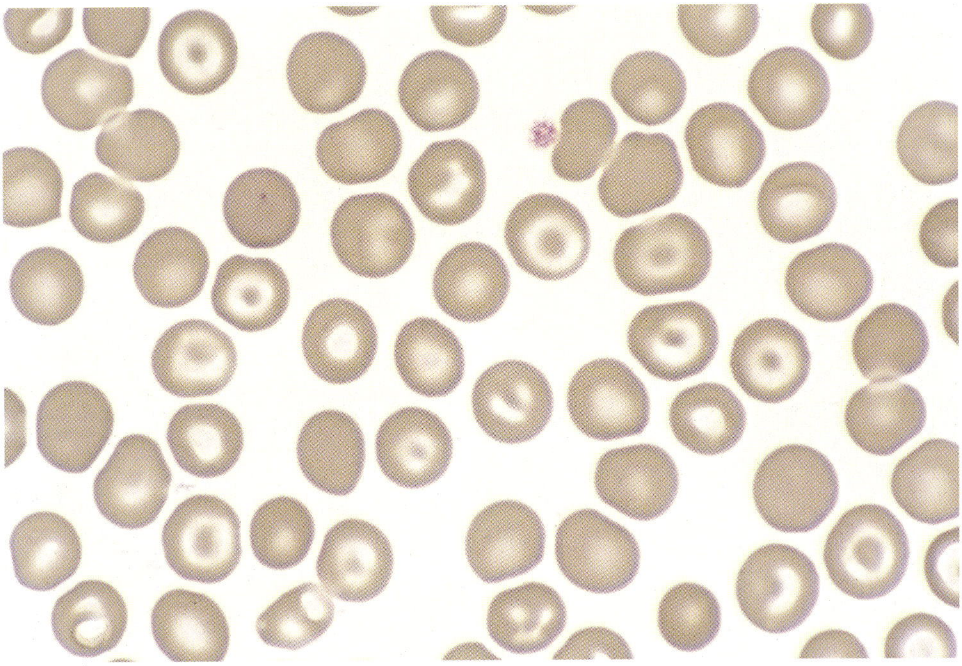

Blood film comments	
Red cell comments	Slight anisocytosis Moderate macrocytes Moderate target cells
White cell comments	Neutrophilia
Platelet comments	Thrombocytopenia

Question 1. What is the differential diagnosis?

Based on the differential diagnosis, the following tests should be requested				
Liver function tests				
Bilirubin total	20	μmol/L	RR (0–25)	μmol/L
ALP	53	U/L	RR (38–126)	U/L
ALT	68	U/L	RR (<45)	U/L
AST	77	U/L	RR (<45)	U/L
GGT	282	U/L	RR (0–50)	U/L

Question 2. Are further tests indicated as part of your final report? If so, which tests?

CASE STUDY 7

Case history

A 59-year-old man with oesophageal varices.

Analyser data				
Parameters	**Test Results**		**Reference Range**	
RBC	2.75	$\times 10^{12}$/L	4.50–6.50	$\times 10^{12}$/L
Hb	76	g/L	130–180	g/L
HCT	0.225		0.40–0.54	
MCV	95.6	fL	80–100	fL
MCH	32.3	pg	26.5–33.0	pg
MCHC	348	g/L	310–360	g/L
RDW-SD	49.8	fL	38.0–48.0	fL
RDW-CV	16.3	%	12.0–14.5	%
RETIC CT				
RETIC ABS				
WBC	7.4	$\times 10^9$/L	3.5–11.0	$\times 10^9$/L
Plat	25	$\times 10^9$/L	150–400	$\times 10^9$/L

Differential						
Parameters	**Test Results**				**Reference Range**	
Neutrophil	63.7	%	4.7	$\times 10^9$/L	1.7–7.0	$\times 10^9$/L
Lymphocyte	22.0	%	1.6	$\times 10^9$/L	1.5–4.0	$\times 10^9$/L
Monocyte	9.7	%	0.7	$\times 10^9$/L	0.1–0.8	$\times 10^9$/L
Eosinophil	3.5	%	0.26	$\times 10^9$/L	0.04–0.44	$\times 10^9$/L
Basophil	1.1	%	0.08	$\times 10^9$/L	0.00–0.20	$\times 10^9$/L

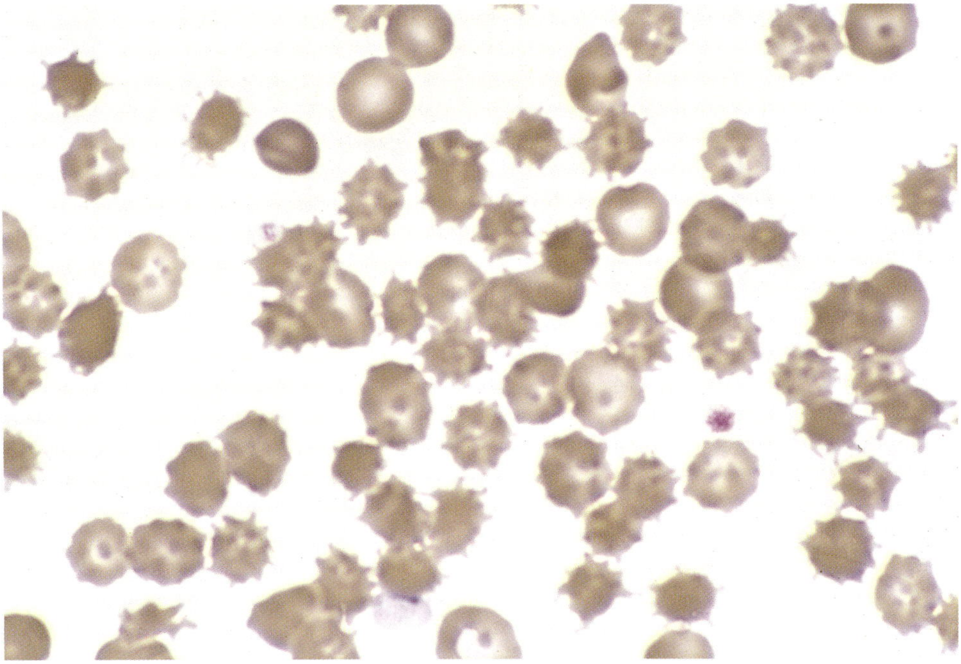

Blood film comments	
Red cell comments	Slight anisocytosis Slight macrocytes Marked spur cells
White cell comments	Normal in number and morphology
Platelet comments	Thrombocytopenia

Question 1. What is the differential diagnosis?

Based on the differential diagnosis, the following tests should be requested				
Liver function tests				
Bilirubin total	10	μmol/L	RR (0–25)	μmol/L
ALP	25	U/L	RR (38–126)	U/L
ALT	28	U/L	RR (<45)	U/L
AST	32	U/L	RR (<45)	U/L
GGT	10	U/L	RR (0–50)	U/L

Question 2. Are further tests indicated as part of your final report? If so, which tests?

CASE STUDY 8

Case history

A 29-year-old female presents with anaemia, and is passing dark urine.

Analyser data				
Parameters	**Test Results**		**Reference Range**	
RBC	2.20	$\times 10^{12}$/L	3.80–5.80	$\times 10^{12}$/L
Hb	76	g/L	115–165	g/L
HCT	0.225		0.37–0.47	
MCV	113.6	fL	80–100	fL
MCH	34.5	pg	26.5–33.0	pg
MCHC	30.4	g/L	310–360	g/L
RDW-SD	76.3	fL	38.0–48.0	fL
RDW-CV	18.2	%	12.0–14.5	%
RETIC CT	16.2	%	0.2–2.0	%
RETIC ABS	356	$\times 10^9$/L	20–80	$\times 10^9$/L
WBC	3.1	$\times 10^9$/L	3.5–11.0	$\times 10^9$/L
Plat	55	$\times 10^9$/L	150–400	$\times 10^9$/L

Differential						
Parameters	**Test Results**				**Reference Range**	
Neutrophil	61.3	%	1.9	$\times 10^9$/L	1.7–7.0	$\times 10^9$/L
Lymphocyte	30.6	%	0.9	$\times 10^9$/L	1.5–4.0	$\times 10^9$/L
Monocyte	6.8	%	0.2	$\times 10^9$/L	0.1–0.8	$\times 10^9$/L
Eosinophil	1.0	%	0.03	$\times 10^9$/L	0.04–0.44	$\times 10^9$/L
Basophil	0.3	%	0.01	$\times 10^9$/L	0.00–0.20	$\times 10^9$/L

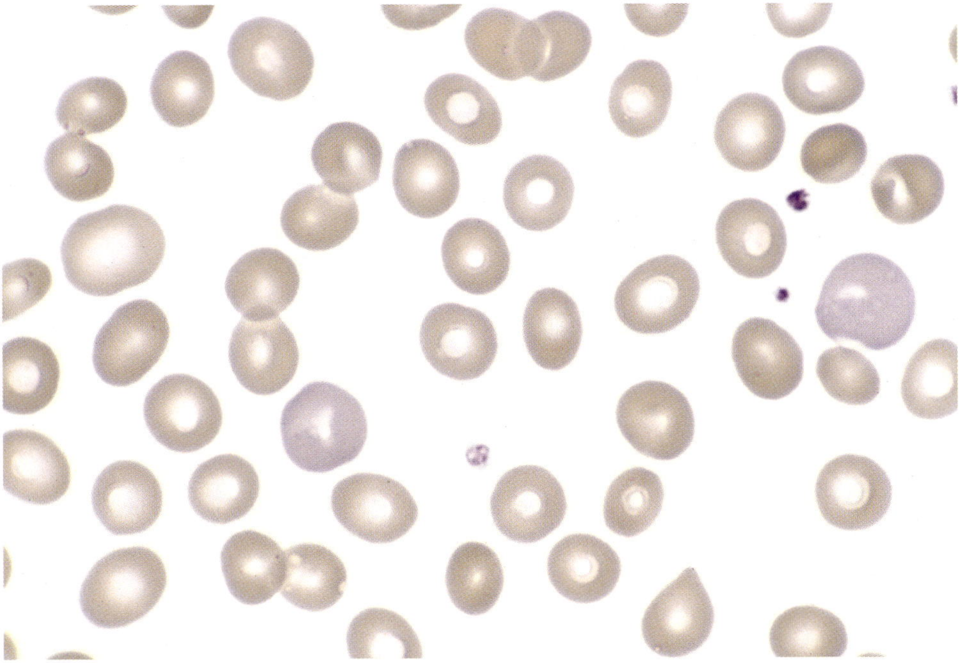

Blood film comments	
Red cell comments	Moderate anisocytosis Moderate macrocytes Marked polychromasia
White cell comments	Lymphopenia
Platelet comments	Thrombocytopenia

Question 1. What is the differential diagnosis?

Based on the differential diagnosis, the following tests should be requested
In paroxysmal nocturnal haemoglobinuria, CD59 expression should be determined on the red cells. In the myeloid lineage, CD33 positivity should be determined followed by expression of CD24/FLAER on the granulocytes and expression of CD14/FLAER on the monocytes.
Flow cytometry CD59 expressed on 100% of the red cells CD24/FLAER expressed on 95% of the granulocytes CD14/FLAER expressed on 95% of the monocytes

Question 2. Are further tests indicated as part of your final report? If so, which tests?

CASE STUDY 9

Case history

A 22-year-old female presents with a history of gall stones.

Analyser data				
Parameters	**Test Results**		**Reference Range**	
RBC	3.87	$\times 10^{12}$/L	3.80–5.80	$\times 10^{12}$/L
Hb	134	g/L	115–165	g/L
HCT	0.402		0.37–0.47	
MCV	91	fL	80–100	fL
MCH	34.6	pg	26.5–33.0	pg
MCHC	371	g/L	310–360	g/L
RDW-SD	48.9	fL	38.0–48.0	fL
RDW-CV	14.8	%	12.0–14.5	%
RETIC CT				
RETIC ABS				
WBC	8.4	$\times 10^9$/L	3.5–11.0	$\times 10^9$/L
Plat	377	$\times 10^9$/L	150–400	$\times 10^9$/L

Differential						
Parameters	**Test Results**				**Reference Range**	
Neutrophil	78.6	%	6.6	$\times 10^9$/L	1.7–7.0	$\times 10^9$/L
Lymphocyte	17.1	%	1.4	$\times 10^9$/L	1.5–4.0	$\times 10^9$/L
Monocyte	3.5	%	0.3	$\times 10^9$/L	0.1–0.8	$\times 10^9$/L
Eosinophil	0.6	%	0.05	$\times 10^9$/L	0.04–0.44	$\times 10^9$/L
Basophil	0.2	%	0.02	$\times 10^9$/L	0.00–0.20	$\times 10^9$/L

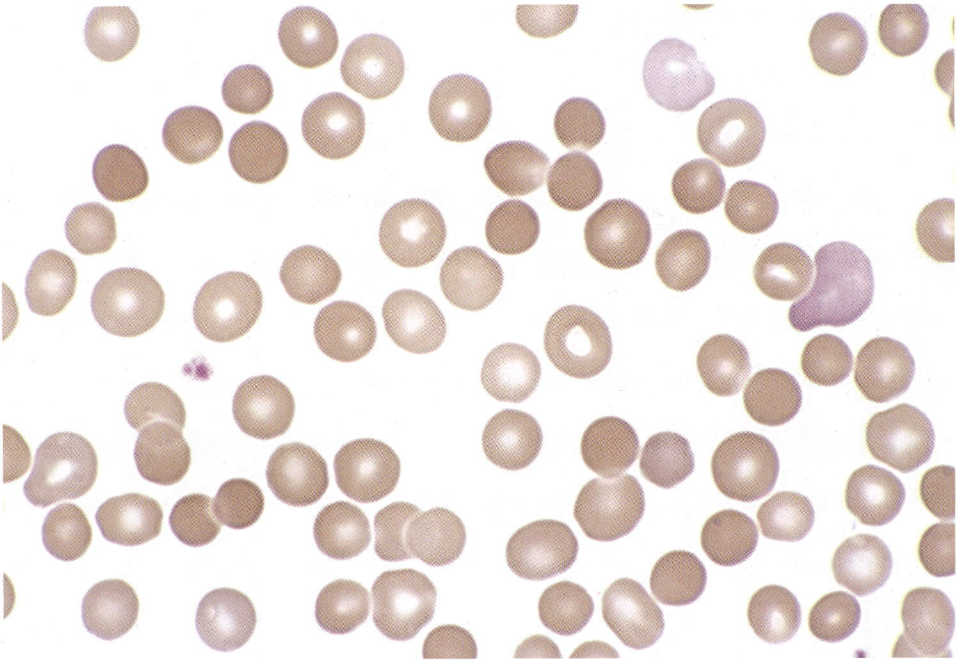

Blood film comments	
Red cell comments	Slight anisocytosis Slight polychromasia Moderate spherocytes
White cell comments	Normal in number and morphology
Platelet comments	Normal in number and morphology

Question 1. What is the differential diagnosis?

Based on the differential diagnosis, the following tests should be requested				
Reticulocyte count				
Reticulocyte count	4.2	%	RR (0.2–2.0)	%
Reticulocyte abs.	162.5	$\times 10^9$/L	RR (20–80)	$\times 10^9$/L
Direct antiglobulin test (DAT): Negative				

The eosin 5 maleimide (EMA) binding by flow cytometry: Reduced.

Question 2. Are further tests indicated as part of your final report? If so, which tests?

CASE STUDY 10

Case history

A 4-year-old female presents with an acute episode of jaundice.

Analyser data				
Parameters	**Test Results**		**Reference Range**	
RBC	1.80	$\times 10^{12}/L$	3.86–5.01	$\times 10^{12}/L$
Hb	56	g/L	107–136	g/L
HCT	0.167		0.31–0.38	
MCV	93.9	fL	73–85	fL
MCH	31.1	pg	24.8–29.9	pg
MCHC	331	g/L	310–360	g/L
RDW-SD	54.5	fL	34.3–44.1	fL
RDW-CV	15.8	%	12.1–15.6	%
RETIC CT				
RETIC ABS				
WBC	31.8	$\times 10^9/L$	4.9–12.8	$\times 10^9/L$
Plat	197	$\times 10^9/L$	214–483	$\times 10^9/L$

Differential						
Parameters	**Test Results**				**Reference Range**	
Neutrophil	58.0	%	18.4	$\times 10^9/L$	1.7–6.7	$\times 10^9/L$
Lymphocyte	26.0	%	8.3	$\times 10^9/L$	2.0–6.6	$\times 10^9/L$
Monocyte	3.0	%	0.1	$\times 10^9/L$	0.2–1.0	$\times 10^9/L$
Eosinophil	2.0	%	0.64	$\times 10^9/L$	0.00–0.60	$\times 10^9/L$
Basophil	0.0	%	0.00	$\times 10^9/L$	0.00–0.10	$\times 10^9/L$
Metamyelocyte	5	%				
Myelocyte	2	%				
Band form	4	%				
NRBC	53 / 100 WBC					

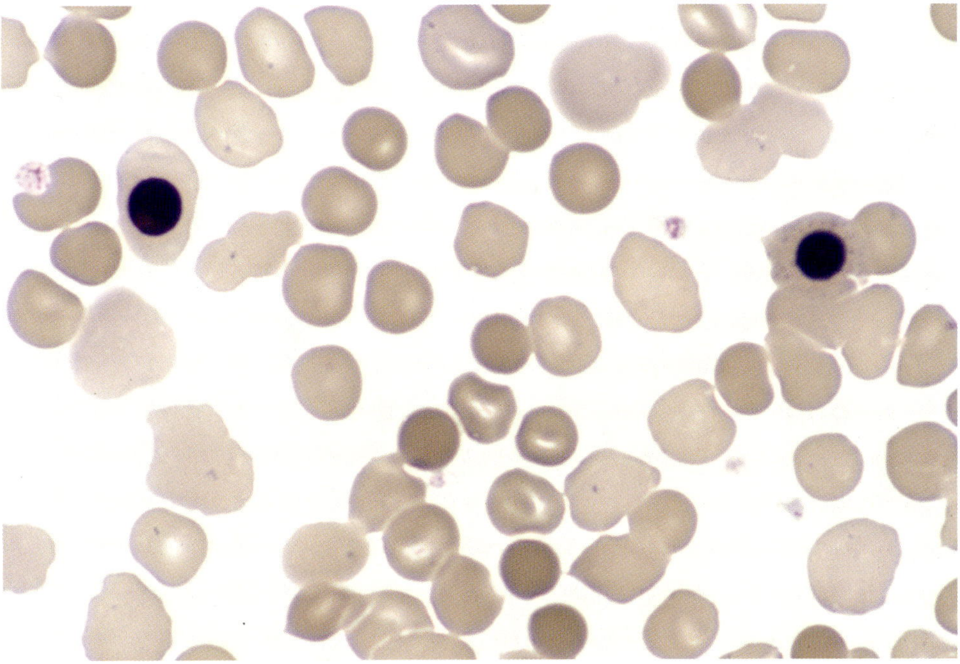

Blood film comments	
Red cell comments	Slight anisocytosis Marked polychromasia Moderate spherocytes 53 NRBC / 100 WBC
White cell comments	Left shift in the myeloid line Neutrophilia
Platelet comments	Normal in number and morphology

Question 1. What is the differential diagnosis?

Based on the differential diagnosis, the following tests should be requested				
Reticulocyte count				
Reticulocyte count	18.1	%	RR (0.2–2.0)	%
Reticulocyte Abs.	325.8	$\times 10^9/L$	RR (20–80)	$\times 10^9/L$
Direct antiglobulin test (DAT): Positive (IgG)				

Question 2. Are further tests indicated as part of your final report? If so, which tests?

CASE STUDY 11

Case history

A newborn with unexplained jaundice.

Analyser data

Parameters	Test Results		Reference Range	
RBC	3.62	× 10^{12}/L	3.34–5.40	× 10^{12}/L
Hb	136	g/L	121–191	g/L
HCT	0.453		0.37–0.60	
MCV	111.0	fL	101–117	fL
MCH	37.6	pg	33.0–38.0	pg
MCHC	338	g/L	310–360	g/L
RDW-SD	75.2	fL	61.9–81.4	fL
RDW-CV	16.4	%	15.5–19.2	%
RETIC CT	6.5	%	4.0–7.0	%
RETIC ABS	235.3	× 10^9/L		
WBC	13.0	× 10^9/L	9.6–30.4	× 10^9/L
Plat	348	× 10^9/L	195–434	× 10^9/L

Differential

Parameters	Test Results				Reference Range	
Neutrophil	68.0	%	8.8	× 10^9/L	4.4–21.0	× 10^9/L
Lymphocyte	24.0	%	3.1	× 10^9/L	2.5–9.1	× 10^9/L
Monocyte	4.0	%	0.5	× 10^9/L	0.6–4.1	× 10^9/L
Eosinophil	4.0	%	0.52	× 10^9/L	0.00–1.30	× 10^9/L
Basophil	0.0	%	0.00	× 10^9/L	0.00–0.40	× 10^9/L
NRBC	31 / 100 WBC				1–25	

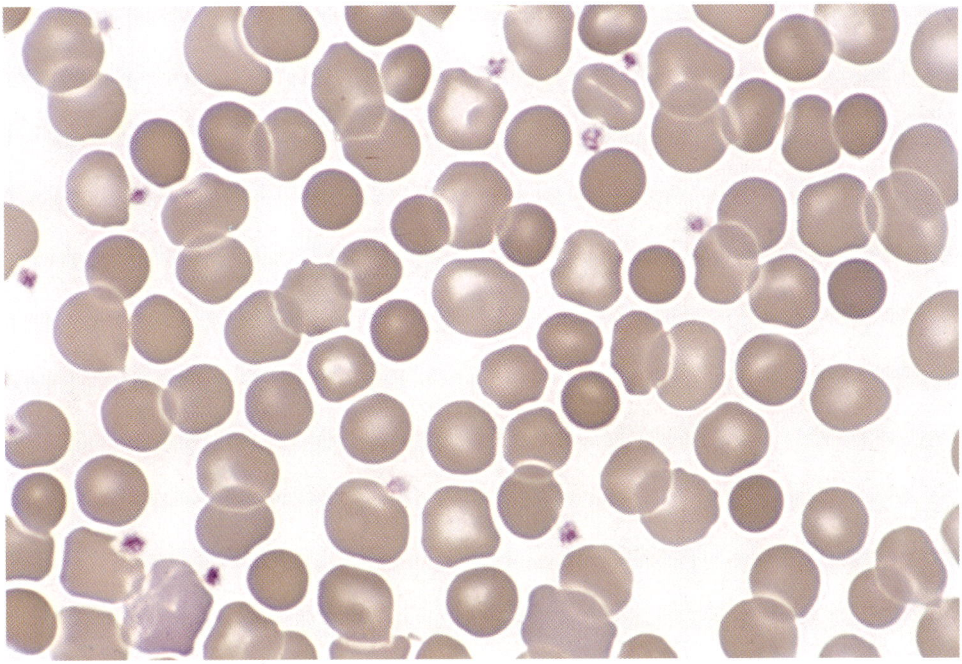

Blood film comments	
Red cell comments	Slight anisocytosis Moderate macrocytes Moderate polychromasia Moderate spherocytes 31 NRBC / 100 WBC
White cell comments	Normal in number and morphology
Platelet comments	Normal in number and morphology

Question 1. What is the differential diagnosis?

Based on the differential diagnosis, the following tests should be requested	
Blood group on the mother Blood group on the neonate DAT	Blood group O Blood group A Negative
The mother will be group O and the neonate group A or group B. The DAT is negative; however, it may be weakly positive. It is highly unlikely the baby will be born with hereditary spherocytosis unless one or both of the parents have hereditary spherocytosis. See Figure A5-1 in *Microscopic Haematology* 3rd edn, where the parents were first cousins and both had HS.	

Question 2. Are further tests indicated as part of your final report? If so, which tests?

CASE STUDY 12

Case history

A newborn whose mother has a high titre of anti D.

Analyser data				
Parameters	**Test Results**		**Reference Range**	
RBC	3.62	$\times 10^{12}$/L	3.34–5.40	$\times 10^{12}$/L
Hb	120	g/L	121–191	g/L
HCT	0.362		0.37–0.60	
MCV	140	fL	101–117	fL
MCH	41.3	pg	33.0–38.0	pg
MCHC	339	g/L	310–360	g/L
RDW-SD	89.2	fL	61.9–81.4	fL
RDW-CV	19.3	%	15.5–19.2	%
RETIC CT	32.0	%	4.0–7.0	%
RETIC ABS	1158.4	$\times 10^9$/L		
WBC	22.9	$\times 10^9$/L	9.6–30.4	$\times 10^9$/L
Plat	321	$\times 10^9$/L	195–434	$\times 10^9$/L

Differential						
Parameters	**Test Results**				**Reference Range**	
Neutrophil	69.0	%	15.8	$\times 10^9$/L	4.4–21.0	$\times 10^9$/L
Lymphocyte	22.0	%	5.0	$\times 10^9$/L	2.5–9.1	$\times 10^9$/L
Monocyte	9.0	%	2.1	$\times 10^9$/L	0.6–4.1	$\times 10^9$/L
Eosinophil	0.0	%	0.00	$\times 10^9$/L	0.00–1.30	$\times 10^9$/L
Basophil	0.0	%	0.00	$\times 10^9$/L	0.00–0.40	$\times 10^9$/L
NRBC	432 / 100 WBC				1–25	

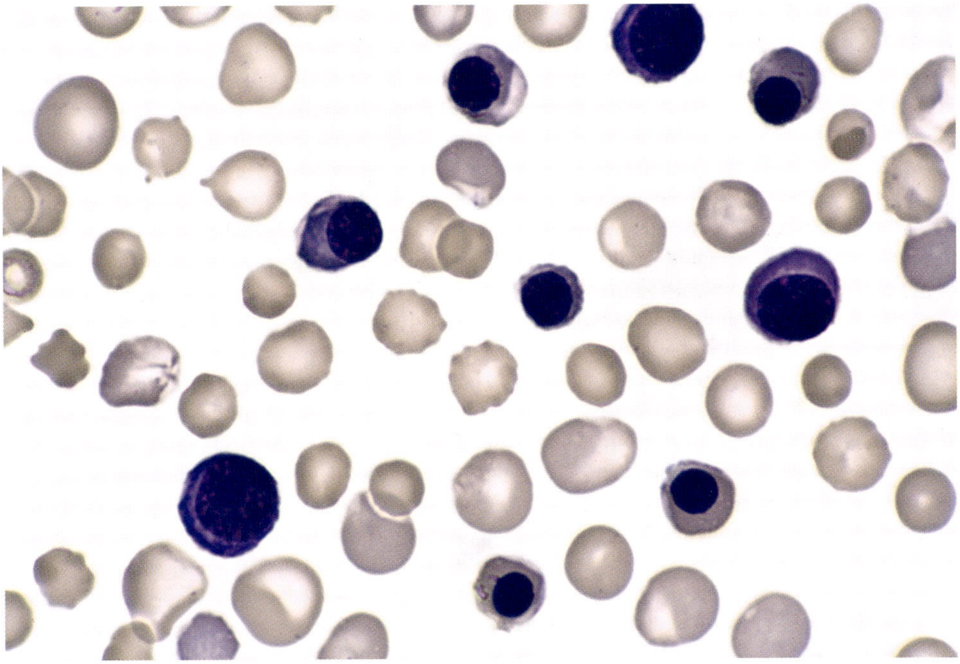

Blood film comments	
Red cell comments	Slight anisocytosis Moderate macrocytes Marked polychromasia 432 NRBC / 100 WBC
White cell comments	Normal in number and morphology
Platelet comments	Normal in number and morphology

Question 1. What is the differential diagnosis?

Based on the differential diagnosis, the following tests should be requested
Direct antiglobulin test (DAT) Strongly positive.

Question 2. Are further tests indicated as part of your final report? If so, which tests?

CASE STUDY 13

Case history

A newborn infant with marked jaundice, anaemia and low MCV for age.

Analyser data

Parameters	**Test Results**		**Reference Range**	
RBC	4.02	$\times 10^{12}$/L	3.34–5.40	$\times 10^{12}$/L
Hb	113	g/L	121–191	g/L
HCT	0.340		0.37–0.60	
MCV	84.6	fL	101–117	fL
MCH	28.1	pg	33.0–38.0	pg
MCHC	332	g/L	310–360	g/L
RDW-SD	83.4	fL	61.9–81.4	fL
RDW-CV	19.2	%	15.5–19.2	%
RETIC CT	15.2	%	4.0–7.0	%
RETIC ABS	611.0	$\times 10^{9}$/L		
WBC	17.4	$\times 10^{9}$/L	9.6–30.4	$\times 10^{9}$/L
Plat	203	$\times 10^{9}$/L	195–434	$\times 10^{9}$/L

Differential

Parameters	**Test Results**				**Reference Range**	
Neutrophil	79.0	%	13.7	$\times 10^{9}$/L	4.4–21.0	$\times 10^{9}$/L
Lymphocyte	2.0	%	0.4	$\times 10^{9}$/L	2.5–9.1	$\times 10^{9}$/L
Monocyte	6.0	%	1.0	$\times 10^{9}$/L	0.6–4.1	$\times 10^{9}$/L
Eosinophil	0.0	%	0.00	$\times 10^{9}$/L	0.00–1.30	$\times 10^{9}$/L
Basophil	0.0	%	0.00	$\times 10^{9}$/L	0.00–0.40	$\times 10^{9}$/L
Band form	6	%				
Metamyelocyte	6	%				
Myelocyte	1	%				
NRBC	31 / 100 WBC				1–25	

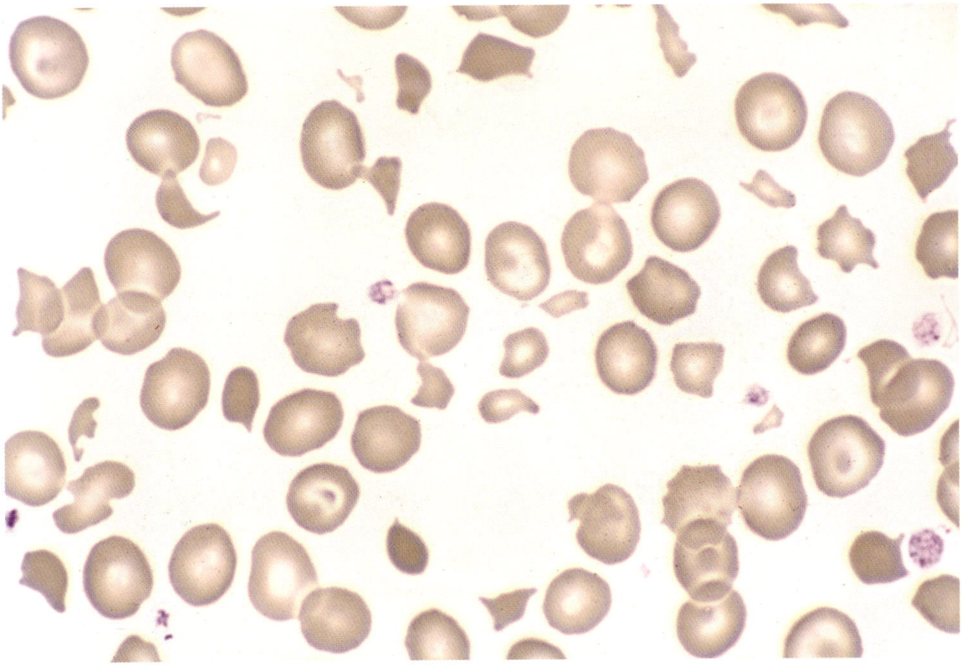

Blood film comments	
Red cell comments	Marked anisocytosis Moderate microcytes Slight macrocytes Moderate polychromasia Slight spherocytes Marked fragments 31 NRBC / 100 WBC
White cell comments	Left shift in the myeloid line.
Platelet comments	Normal in number and morphology. (Note that the increased number of red cell fragments may falsely elevate the platelet count.)

Question 1. What is the differential diagnosis?

Based on the differential diagnosis, the following tests should be requested				
Bilirubin total	375	µmol/L	RR (0–85)	µmol/L
Bilirubin conjugated	249	µmol/L	RR (<10)	µmol/L
The eosin 5 maleimide (EMA) binding by flow cytometry: Reduced				

Question 2. Are further tests indicated as part of your final report? If so, which tests?

CASE STUDY 14

Case history

A 53-year-old female with ovarian cancer presents with severe abdominal pain.

Analyser data				
Parameters	**Test Results**		**Reference Range**	
RBC	2.52	$\times 10^{12}/L$	3.80–5.80	$\times 10^{12}/L$
Hb	76	g/L	115–165	g/L
HCT	0.223		0.37–0.47	
MCV	92.1	fL	80–100	fL
MCH	30.2	pg	26.5–33.0	pg
MCHC	328	g/L	310–360	g/L
RDW-SD	52.1	fL	38.0–48.0	fL
RDW-CV	16.8	%	12.0–14.5	%
RETIC CT				
RETIC ABS				
WBC	15.2	$\times 10^9/L$	3.5–11.0	$\times 10^9/L$
Plat	163	$\times 10^9/$	150–400	$\times 10^9/L$
ESR	87 mm/h		<10 mm/h	

Differential						
Parameters	**Test Results**				**Reference Range**	
Neutrophil	74.4	%	11.3	$\times 10^9/L$	1.7–7.0	$\times 10^9/L$
Lymphocyte	12.8	%	2.0	$\times 10^9/L$	1.5–4.0	$\times 10^9/L$
Monocyte	10.3	%	1.6	$\times 10^9/L$	0.1–0.8	$\times 10^9/L$
Eosinophil	2.0	%	0.31	$\times 10^9/L$	0.04–0.44	$\times 10^9/L$
Basophil	0.5	%	0.07	$\times 10^9/L$	0.00–0.20	$\times 10^9/L$

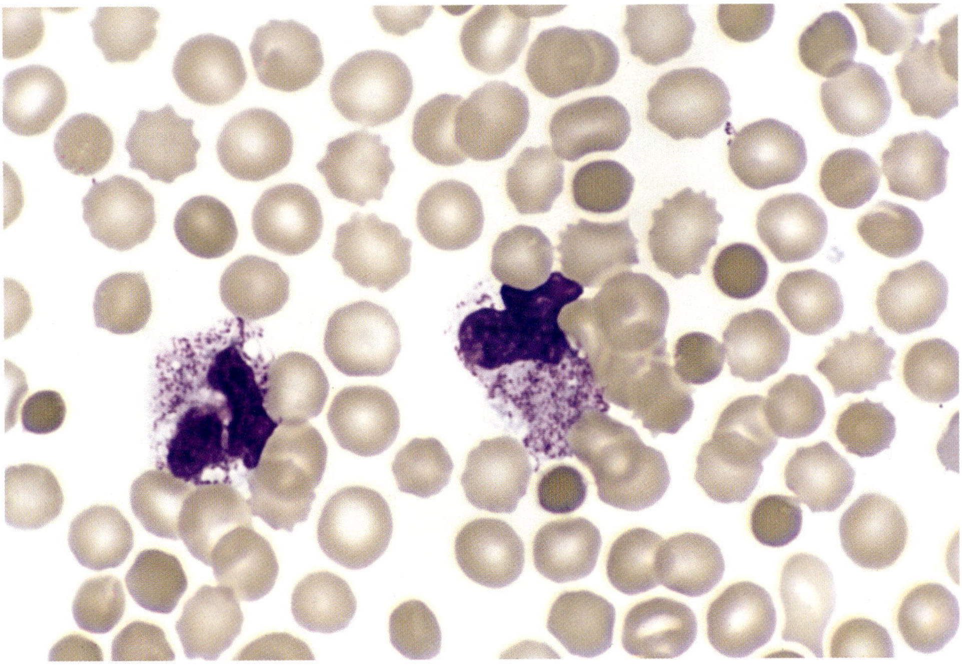

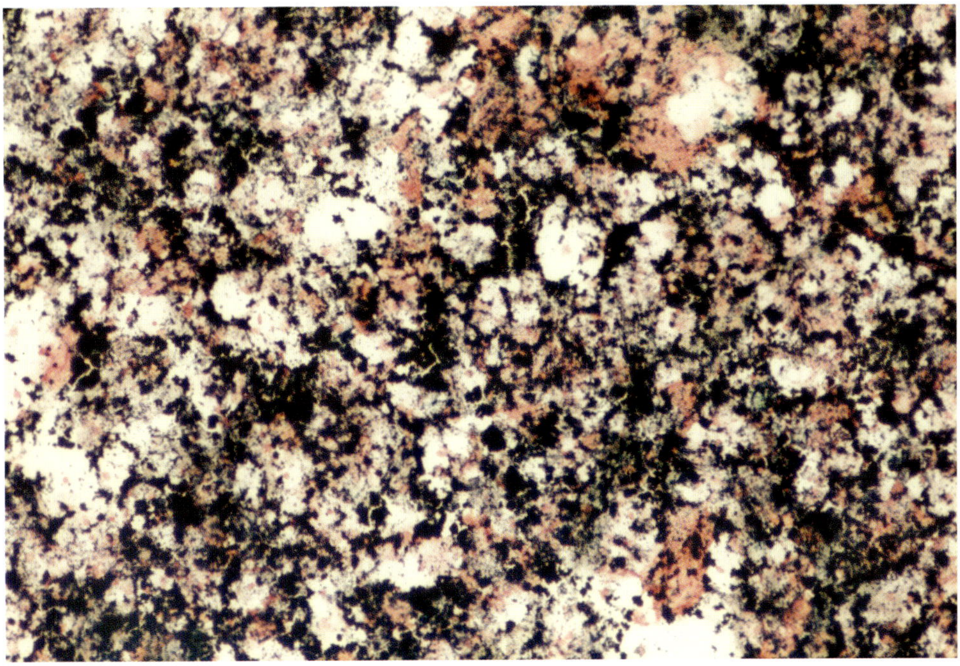

Urinary haemosiderin

Blood film comments	
Red cell comments	Slight anisocytosis Moderate spherocytes Moderate rouleaux
White cell comments	Toxic granulation Neutrophilia
Platelet comments	Normal in number and morphology

Question 1. What is the differential diagnosis?

Based on the differential diagnosis, the following tests should be requested				
Urinary haemosiderin Positive				
Reticulocyte count				
Retic	2.4	%	RR (0.2–2.0)	%
Retic abs.	60.5	× 10^9/L	RR (20–80)	× 10^9/L
Coagulation studies				
PT	23.4	sec	RR (12.0–15.0)	sec
INR	2.1		RR (0.8–1.1)	
APTT	47.1	sec	RR (25.0–35.0)	sec
LD	1936	U/L	RR (90–200)	U/L
Urea	11.1	mmol/L	RR (2.9–7.1)	mmol/L
Creatinine	206	µmol/L	RR (60–110)	µmol/L
Bilirubin (t)	507	µmol/L	RR (0–25)	µmol/L
ALP	48	U/L	RR (38–126)	U/L
GGT	10	U/L	RR (0–30)	U/L
AST	2550	U/L	RR (<45)	U/L
ALT	590	U/L	RR (<45)	U/L

Question 2. Are further tests indicated as part of your final report? If so, which tests?

CASE STUDY 15

Case history

A 3-year-old child presents with bloody diarrhoea.

Analyser data

Parameters	Test Results		Reference Range	
RBC	3.58	× 10^{12}/L	3.86–5.01	× 10^{12}/L
Hb	92	g/L	107–136	g/L
HCT	0.280		0.31–0.38	
MCV	78.5	fL	73–85	fL
MCH	25.7	pg	24.8–29.9	pg
MCHC	327	g/L	310–360	g/L
RDW-SD	48.4	fL	34.3–44.1	fL
RDW-CV	15.1	%	12.1–15.6	%
RETIC CT				
RETIC ABS				
WBC	18.6	× 10^9/L	4.9–12.8	× 10^9/L
Plat	27	× 10^9/L	214–483	× 10^9/L

Differential

Parameters	Test Results				Reference Range	
Neutrophil	62.0	%	11.4	× 10^9/L	1.7–6.7	× 10^9/L
Lymphocyte	28.0	%	5.2	× 10^9/L	2.0–6.6	× 10^9/L
Monocyte	10.0	%	1.9	× 10^9/L	0.2–1.0	× 10^9/L
Eosinophil	0.0	%	0.00	× 10^9/L	0.00–0.60	× 10^9/L
Basophil	0.0	%	0.00	× 10^9/L	0.00–0.10	× 10^9/L

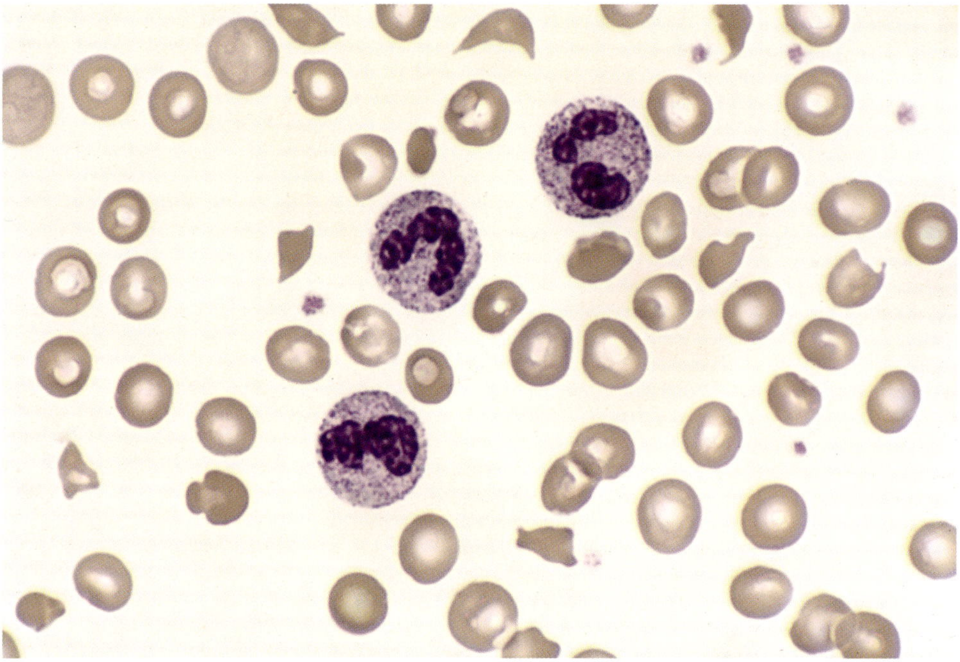

Blood film comments	
Red cell comments	Slight anisocytosis Slight polychromasia Moderate schistocytes
White cell comments	Toxic granulation Neutrophilia
Platelet comments	Thrombocytopenia

Question 1. What is the differential diagnosis?

Based on the differential diagnosis, the following tests should be requested				
Urea	21.5	mmol/L	RR (2.9–7.1)	mmol/L
Creatinine	278	μmol/L	RR (20–40)	μmol/L

Question 2. Are further tests indicated as part of your final report? If so, which tests?

CASE STUDY 16

Case history

A 6-year-old male presents with vomiting and is disorientated.

Analyser data

Parameters	Test Results		Reference Range	
RBC	2.98	$\times 10^{12}$/L	3.96–4.92	$\times 10^{12}$/L
Hb	79	g/L	110–139	g/L
HCT	0.237		0.32–0.39	
MCV	78.5	fL	74–86	fL
MCH	26.5	pg	25.5–30.6	pg
MCHC	338	g/L	310–360	g/L
RDW-SD	39.1	fL	34.6–42.7	fL
RDW-CV	13.9	%	11.9–14.9	%
RETIC CT				
RETIC ABS				
WBC	19.8	$\times 10^9$/L	4.7–12.3	$\times 10^9$/L
Plat	36	$\times 10^9$/L	205–457	$\times 10^9$/L

Differential

Parameters	Test Results				Reference Range	
Neutrophil	64.0	%	12.7	$\times 10^9$/L	1.8–7.7	$\times 10^9$/L
Lymphocyte	4.0	%	0.8	$\times 10^9$/L	1.6–5.1	$\times 10^9$/L
Monocyte	5.0	%	0.9	$\times 10^9$/L	0.1–1.0	$\times 10^9$/L
Eosinophil	0.0	%	0.00	$\times 10^9$/L	0.00–0.60	$\times 10^9$/L
Basophil	0.0	%	0.00	$\times 10^9$/L	1.00–0.10	$\times 10^9$/L

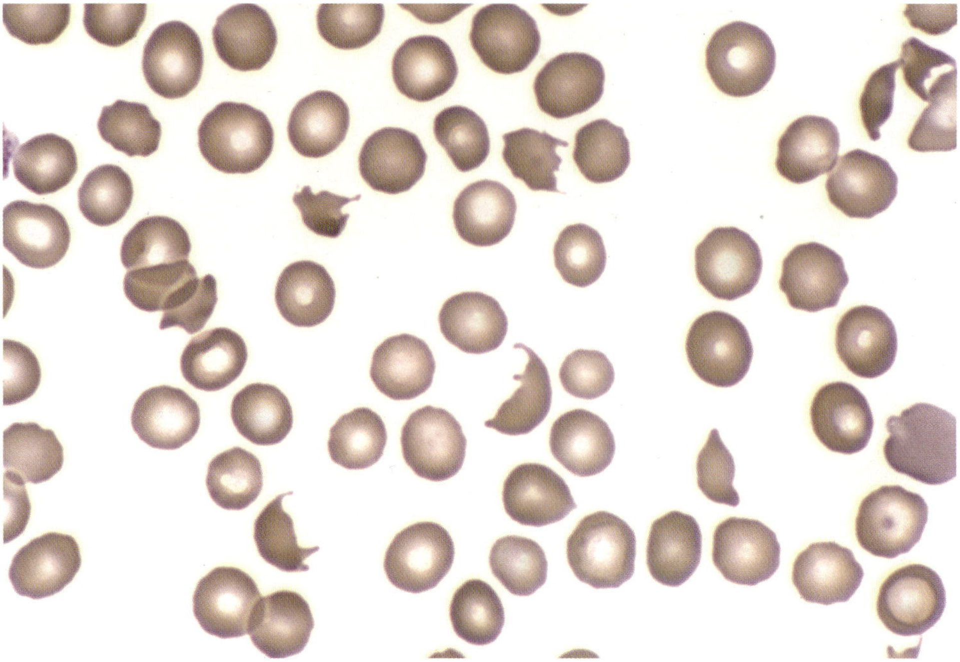

Blood film comments	
Red cell comments	Slight polychromasia Moderate schistocytes
White cell comments	Neutrophilia Lymphopenia
Platelet comments	Marked thrombocytopenia

Question 1. What is the differential diagnosis?

Based on the differential diagnosis, the following tests should be requested				
Urea	23.9	mmol/L	RR (2.9–7.1)	mmol/L
Creatinine	195	μmol/L	RR (30–60)	μmol/L

Question 2. Are further tests indicated as part of your final report? If so, which tests?

CASE STUDY 17

Case history

A 72-year-old male with a prosthetic heart valve.

Analyser data

Parameters	Test Results		Reference Range	
RBC	2.44	× 10^{12}/L	4.50–6.50	× 10^{12}/L
Hb	78	g/L	130–180	g/L
HCT	0.236		0.40–0.54	
MCV	95.5	fL	80–100	fL
MCH	32.0	pg	26.5–33.0	pg
MCHC	335	g/L	310–360	g/L
RDW-SD	50.1	fL	38.0–48.0	fL
RDW-CV	15.6	%	12.0–14.5	%
RETIC CT				
RETIC ABS				
WBC	12.2	× 10^9/L	3.5–11.0	× 10^9/L
Plat	242	× 10^9/L	150–400	× 10^9/L

Differential

Parameters	Test Results				Reference Range	
Neutrophil	80.7	%	9.8	× 10^9/L	1.7–7.0	× 10^9/L
Lymphocyte	11.5	%	1.4	× 10^9/L	1.5–4.0	× 10^9/L
Monocyte	5.5	%	0.7	× 10^9/L	0.1–0.8	× 10^9/L
Eosinophil	1.6	%	0.19	× 10^9/L	0.04–0.44	× 10^9/L
Basophil	0.7	%	0.08	× 10^9/L	0.00–0.20	× 10^9/L

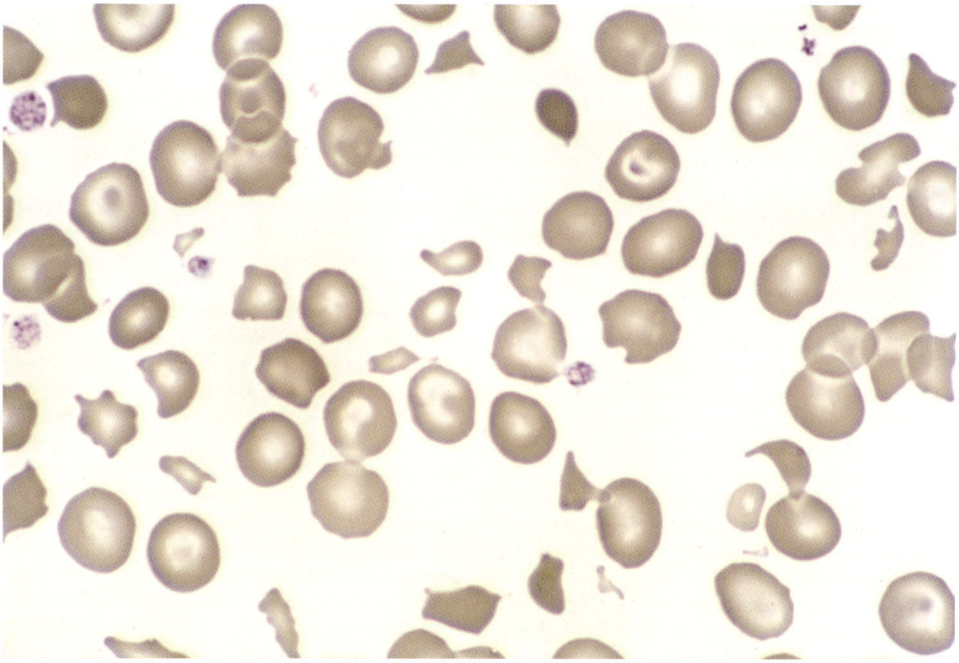

Blood film comments	
Red cell comments	Slight anisocytosis Moderate polychromasia Moderate schistocytes
White cell comments	Neutrophilia
Platelet comments	Normal in number and morphology (Note that the increased number of schistocytes may falsely elevate the platelet count.)

Question 1. What is the differential diagnosis?

Based on the differential diagnosis, the following tests should be requested				
Reticulocyte count				
Retic	7.3	%	RR (0.2–2.0)	%
Retic abs.	178.1	× 10^9/L	RR (20–80)	× 10^9/L
LDH	406	U/L	RR (90–200)	U/L

Question 2. Are further tests indicated as part of your final report? If so, which tests?

CASE STUDY 18

Case history

A 33-year-old female presents in the third trimester of pregnancy with toxaemia.

Analyser data				
Parameters	**Test Results**		**Reference Range**	
RBC	4.23	$\times 10^{12}/L$	3.80–5.80	$\times 10^{12}/L$
Hb	127	g/L	115–165	g/L
HCT	0.381		0.37–0.47	
MCV	85.6	fL	80–100	fL
MCH	30.0	pg	26.5–33.0	pg
MCHC	351	g/L	310–360	g/L
RDW-SD	48.7	fL	38.0–48.0	fL
RDW-CV	14.9	%	12.0–14.5	%
RETIC CT				
RETIC ABS				
WBC	17.5	$\times 10^9/L$	3.5–11.0	$\times 10^9/L$
Plat	89	$\times 10^9/L$	150–400	$\times 10^9/L$

Differential						
Parameters	**Test Results**				**Reference Range**	
Neutrophil	93.5	%	16.4	$\times 10^9/L$	1.7–7.0	$\times 10^9/L$
Lymphocyte	3.5	%	0.6	$\times 10^9/L$	1.5–4.0	$\times 10^9/L$
Monocyte	2.7	%	0.5	$\times 10^9/L$	0.1–0.8	$\times 10^9/L$
Eosinophil	0.2	%	0.03	$\times 10^9/L$	0.04–0.44	$\times 10^9/L$
Basophil	0.1	%	0.01	$\times 10^9/L$	0.00–0.20	$\times 10^9/L$

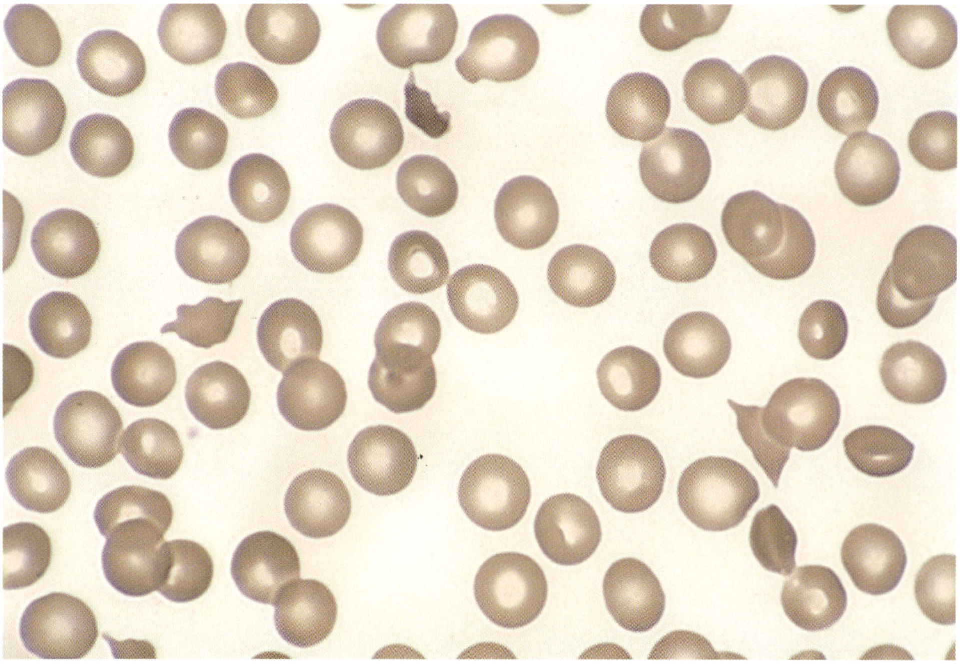

Blood film comments	
Red cell comments	Slight anisocytosis Slight schistocytes
White cell comments	Neutrophilia
Platelet comments	Thrombocytopenia

Question 1. What is the differential diagnosis?

Based on the differential diagnosis, the following tests should be requested				
Urea	10.1	mmol/L	RR (2.9–7.1)	mmol/L
Creatinine	132	μmol/L	RR (60–110)	μmol/L
Bilirubin (t)	30	μmol/L	RR (0–25)	μmol/L
ALP	238	U/L	RR (38–126)	U/L
GGT	57	U/L	RR (0–30)	U/L
AST	224	U/L	RR (<45)	U/L
ALT	385	U/L	RR (<45)	U/L

Question 2. Are further tests indicated as part of your final report? If so, which tests?

CASE STUDY 19

Case history

A 3-weeks-old 34/40 premature neonate with jaundice and a drop in haemoglobin.

Analyser data				
Parameters	**Test Results**		**Reference Range**	
RBC	3.00	$\times 10^{12}$/L	3.38–3.94	$\times 10^{12}$/L
Hb	93	g/L	102–130	g/L
HCT	0.279		0.30–0.38	
MCV	97.7	fL	84–98	fL
MCH	31.0	pg	29.0–33.8	pg
MCHC	317	g/L	310–360	g/L
RDW-SD	51.2	fL	39.9–56.6	fL
RDW-CV	18.2	%	12.6–16.0	%
RETIC CT	12.6	%	0.2–2.0	%
RETIC ABS	378	$\times 10^9$/L	20–80	$\times 10^9$/L
WBC	13.8	$\times 10^9$/L	6.4–12.1	$\times 10^9$/L
Plat	392	$\times 10^9$/L	270–645	$\times 10^9$/L

Differential						
Parameters	**Test Results**				**Reference Range**	
Neutrophil	46	%	6.3	$\times 10^9$/L	0.8–4.9	$\times 10^9$/L
Lymphocyte	36	%	5.0	$\times 10^9$/L	3.8–7.6	$\times 10^9$/L
Monocyte	9.0	%	1.2	$\times 10^9$/L	0.3–1.2	$\times 10^9$/L
Eosinophil	9.0	%	1.20	$\times 10^9$/L	0.10–0.80	$\times 10^9$/L
Basophil	0.0	%	0.00	$\times 10^9$/L	0.00–0.20	$\times 10^9$/L
NRBC	10 / 100 WBC				1–25	

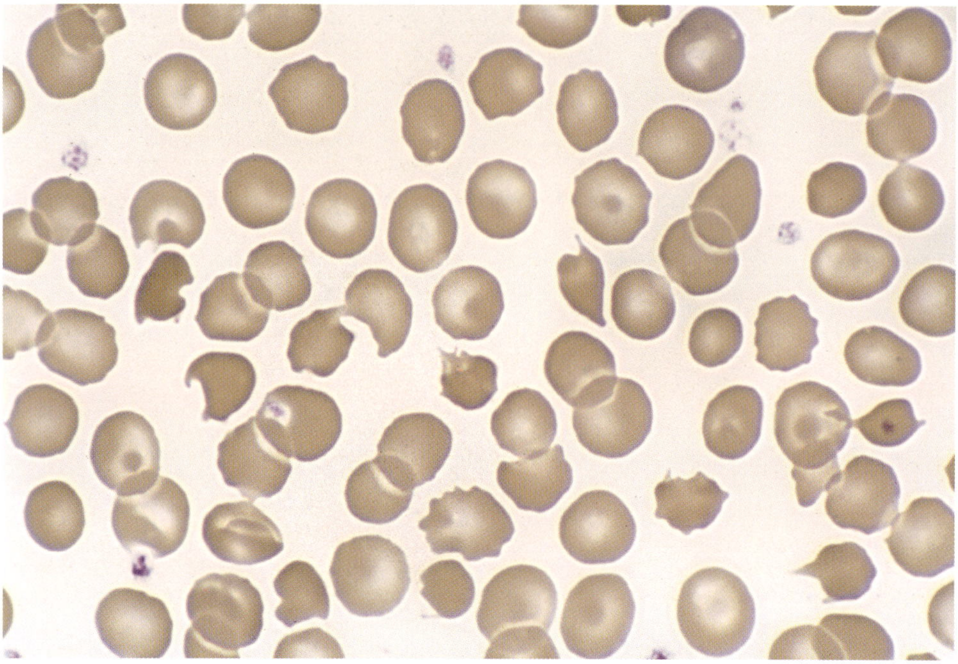

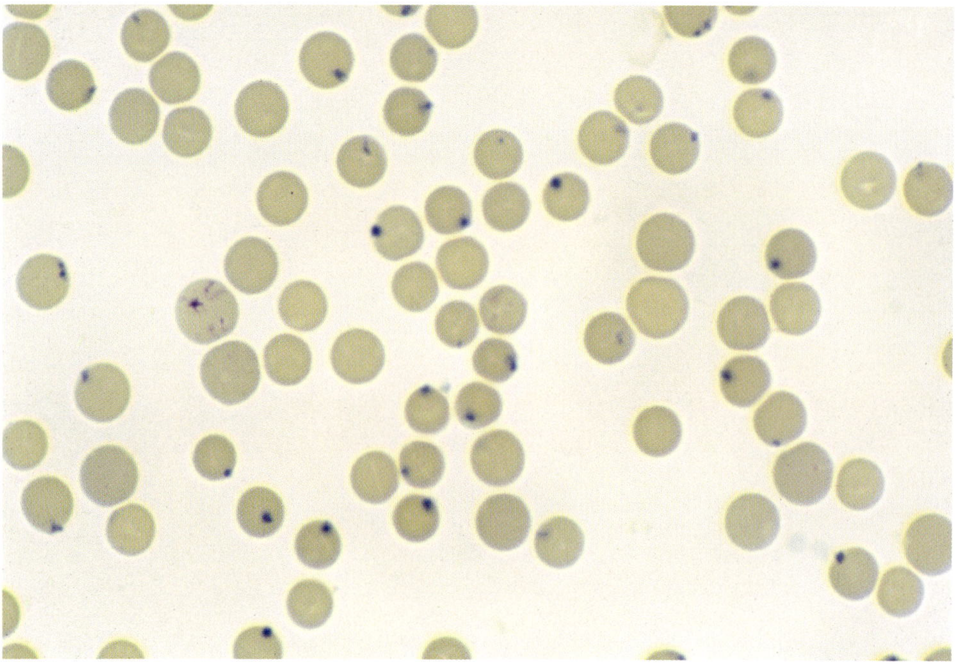

Heinz bodies in a splenectomised adult (cresyl blue stain)

Blood film comments	
Red cell comments	Slight anisocytosis Slight macrocytes Moderate polychromasia Moderate bite cells 10 NRBC / 100 WBC
White cell comments	Neutrophilia Eosinophilia
Platelet comments	Normal in number and morphology

Question 1. What is the differential diagnosis?

Based on the differential diagnosis, the following tests should be requested
G6PD screen / G6PD assay G6PD screen: normal activity.

Question 2. Are further tests indicated as part of your final report? If so, which tests?

CASE STUDY 20

Case history
A 25-year-old female of Asian origin and four weeks pregnant.

Analyser data				
Parameters	**Test Results**		**Reference Range**	
RBC	5.25	$\times 10^{12}$/L	3.80–5.80	$\times 10^{12}$/L
Hb	108	g/L	115–165	g/L
HCT	0.324		0.37–0.47	
MCV	65.0	fL	80–100	fL
MCH	20.6	pg	26.5–33.0	pg
MCHC	317	g/L	310–360	g/L
RDW-SD	33.9	fL	38.0–48.0	fL
RDW-CV	14.5	%	12.0–14.5	%
RETIC CT				
RETIC ABS				
WBC	9.4	$\times 10^9$/L	3.5–11.0	$\times 10^9$/L
Plat	172	$\times 10^9$/L	150–400	$\times 10^9$/L

Differential						
Parameters	**Test Results**				**Reference Range**	
Neutrophil	60.8	%	5.7	$\times 10^9$/L	1.7–7.0	$\times 10^9$/L
Lymphocyte	23.1	%	2.2	$\times 10^9$/L	1.5–4.0	$\times 10^9$/L
Monocyte	10.0	%	0.9	$\times 10^9$/L	0.1–0.8	$\times 10^9$/L
Eosinophil	5.6	%	0.53	$\times 10^9$/L	0.04–0.44	$\times 10^9$/L
Basophil	0.5	%	0.05	$\times 10^9$/L	0.00–0.20	$\times 10^9$/L

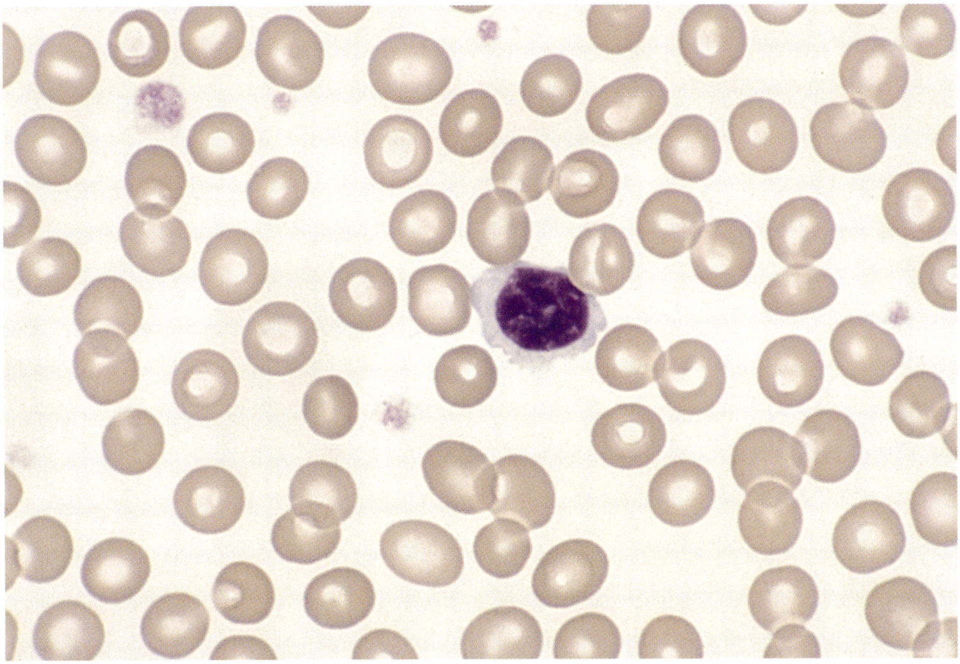

Blood film comments	
Red cell comments	Moderate microcytes Moderate hypochromasia
White cell comments	Eosinophilia
Platelet comments	Normal in number and morphology

Question 1. What is the differential diagnosis?

Based on the differential diagnosis, the following tests should be requested				
Haemoglobin electrophoresis (Hb EPG) Hb EPG cellulose acetate (pH 8.6)				
HbA_2	2.7	%	RR (2.0–3.5)	%
HbF	<1	%	RR (<1)	%
HbH inclusions detected.				

Question 2. Are further tests indicated as part of your final report? If so, which tests?

CASE STUDY 21

Case history

A 31-year-old male has a routine full blood count.

Analyser data				
Parameters	**Test Results**		**Reference Range**	
RBC	5.91	× 10^{12}/L	4.50–6.50	× 10^{12}/L
Hb	102	g/L	130–180	g/L
HCT	0.304		0.40–0.54	
MCV	69.2	fL	80–100	fL
MCH	21.7	pg	26.5–33.0	pg
MCHC	313	g/L	310–360	g/L
RDW-SD	45.2	fL	38.0–48.0	fL
RDW-CV	14.3	%	12.0–14.5	%
RETIC CT				
RETIC ABS				
WBC	6.2	× 10^9/L	3.5–11.0	× 10^9/L
Plat	204	× 10^9/L	150–400	× 10^9/L

Differential						
Parameters	**Test Results**				**Reference Range**	
Neutrophil	61.1	%	3.8	× 10^9/L	1.7–7.0	× 10^9/L
Lymphocyte	26.1	%	1.6	× 10^9/L	1.5–4.0	× 10^9/L
Monocyte	9.9	%	0.6	× 10^9/L	0.1–0.8	× 10^9/L
Eosinophil	2.4	%	0.15	× 10^9/L	0.04–0.44	× 10^9/L
Basophil	0.5	%	0.03	× 10^9/L	0.00–0.20	× 10^9/L

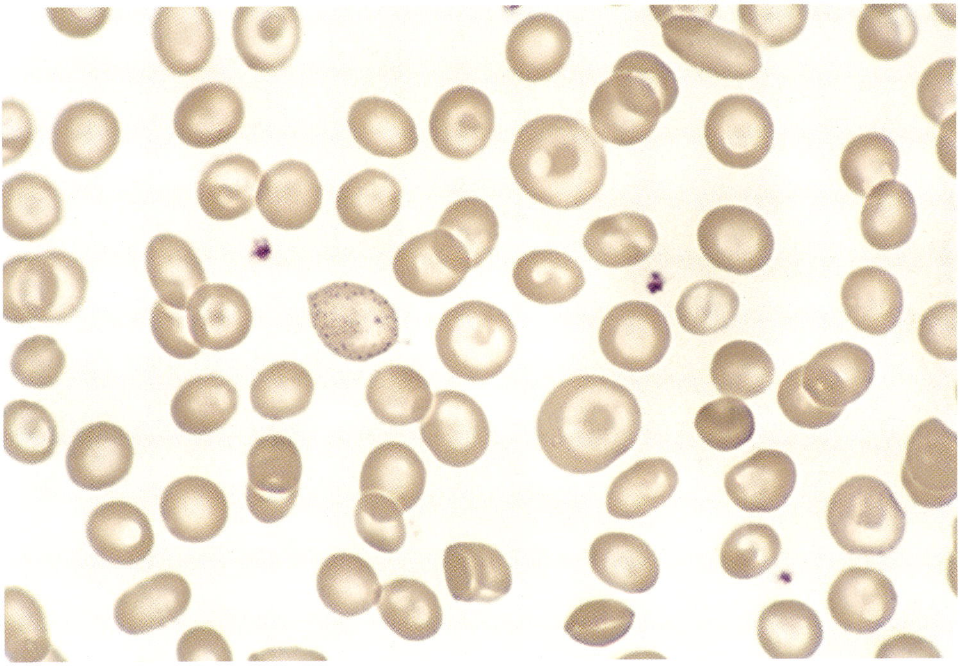

Blood film comments	
Red cell comments	Moderate microcytes Moderate hypochromasia Slight target cells Slight basophilic stippling
White cell comments	Normal in number and morphology
Platelet comments	Normal in number and morphology

Question 1. What is the differential diagnosis?

Based on the differential diagnosis, the following tests should be requested				
Haemoglobin electrophoresis (Hb EPG) Hb EPG cellulose acetate (pH 8.6)				
HbA_2	5.4	%	RR (2.0–3.5)	%
HbF	<1	%	RR (<1)	%
HbH inclusions not detected.				

Question 2. Are further tests indicated as part of your final report? If so, which tests?

CASE STUDY 22

Case history

A 23-year-old male immigrant from Southeast Asia.

Analyser data				
Parameters	**Test Results**		**Reference Range**	
RBC	6.39	× 10^{12}/L	4.50–6.50	× 10^{12}/L
Hb	87	g/L	130–180	g/L
HCT	0.297		0.40–0.54	
MCV	54.9	fL	80–100	fL
MCH	16.1	pg	26.5–33.0	pg
MCHC	293	g/L	310–360	g/L
RDW-SD	52.6	fL	38.0–48.0	fL
RDW-CV	15.9	%	12.0–14.5	%
RETIC CT				
RETIC ABS				
WBC	7.4	× 10^9/L	3.5–11.0	× 10^9/L
Plat	218	× 10^9/L	150–400	× 10^9/L

Differential						
Parameters	**Test Results**				**Reference Range**	
Neutrophil	63.7	%	4.7	× 10^9/L	1.7–7.0	× 10^9/L
Lymphocyte	22.0	%	1.6	× 10^9/L	1.5–4.0	× 10^9/L
Monocyte	9.7	%	0.7	× 10^9/L	0.1–0.8	× 10^9/L
Eosinophil	3.5	%	0.26	× 10^9/L	0.04–0.44	× 10^9/L
Basophil	1.1	%	0.08	× 10^9/L	0.00–0.20	× 10^9/L

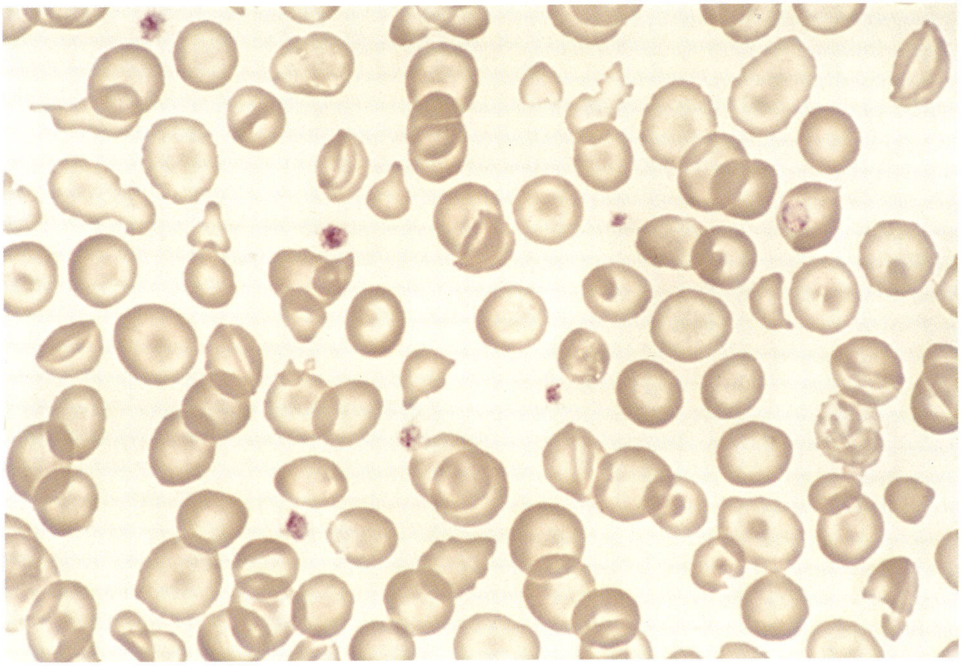

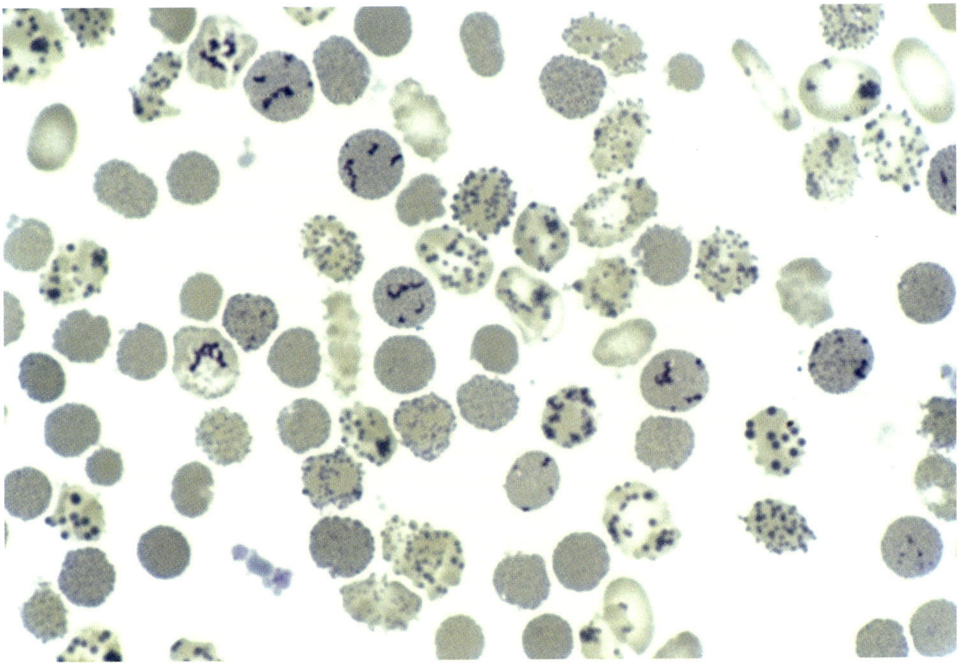

Haemoglobin H preparation (cresyl blue stain)

Blood film comments	
Red cell comments	Slight anisocytosis Moderate microcytes Moderate hypochromasia Slight polychromasia Moderate target cells
White cell comments	Normal in number and morphology
Platelet comments	Normal in number and morphology

Question 1. What is the differential diagnosis?

Based on the differential diagnosis, the following tests should be requested				
Haemoglobin electrophoresis (Hb EPG) Hb EPG cellulose acetate (pH 8.6)				
HbA_2	1.6	%	RR (2.0–3.5)	%
HbF	<1	%	RR (<1)	%
Abnormal band detected in the HbH position. HbH inclusion bodies in the majority of the red blood cells.				

Question 2. Are further tests indicated as part of your final report? If so, which tests?

CASE STUDY 23

Case history

A 3-year-old child with pallor and lethargy.

Analyser data

Parameters	Test Results		Reference Range	
RBC	2.56	$\times 10^{12}$/L	3.86–5.01	$\times 10^{12}$/L
Hb	72	g/L	107–136	g/L
HCT	0.210		0.31–0.38	
MCV	77.7	fL	73–85	fL
MCH	28.1	pg	24.8–29.9	pg
MCHC	359	g/L	310–360	g/L
RDW-SD	50.2	fL	34.3–44.1	fL
RDW-CV	15.2	%	12.1–15.6	%
RETIC CT	4.7	%		
RETIC ABS	120.3	$\times 10^9$/L	20–80	$\times 10^9$/L
WBC	8.7	$\times 10^9$/L	4.9–12.8	$\times 10^9$/L
Plat	358	$\times 10^9$/L	214–483	$\times 10^9$/L

Differential

Parameters	Test Results				Reference Range	
Neutrophil	70.6	%	6.2	$\times 10^9$/L	1.7–6.7	$\times 10^9$/L
Lymphocyte	14.0	%	1.2	$\times 10^9$/L	2.0–6.6	$\times 10^9$/L
Monocyte	4.9	%	0.4	$\times 10^9$/L	0.2–1.0	$\times 10^9$/L
Eosinophil	10.0	%	0.87	$\times 10^9$/L	0.00–0.60	$\times 10^9$/L
Basophil	0.5	%	0.04	$\times 10^9$/L	0.00–0.10	$\times 10^9$/L

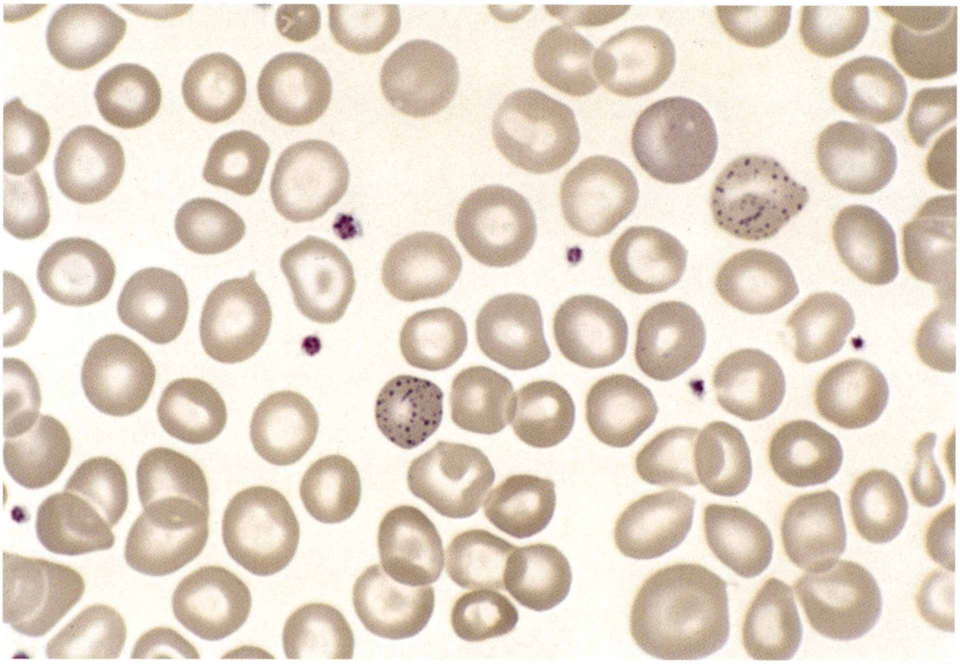

Blood film comments	
Red cell comments	Slight anisocytosis Slight microcytes Slight hypochromasia Slight polychromasia Slight target cells Coarse basophilic stippling
White cell comments	Lymphopenia
Platelet comments	Normal in number and morphology

Question 1. What is the differential diagnosis?

Based on the differential diagnosis, the following tests should be requested				
Haemoglobin electrophoresis (Hb EPG) Hb EPG cellulose acetate (pH 8.6)				
HbA_2	1.4	%	RR (2.0–3.5)	%
HbF	3.3	%	RR (<1)	%
Haemoglobin H inclusions detected in the majority of cells. Abnormal bands detected at HbH and Hb Constant Spring positions. Iron studies are normal.				

Question 2. Are further tests indicated as part of your final report? If so, what?

CASE STUDY 24

Case history

A 39-year-old female feeling lethargic. She is transfusion dependent.

Analyser data				
Parameters	**Test Results**		**Reference Range**	
RBC	4.05	$\times 10^{12}/L$	3.80–5.80	$\times 10^{12}/L$
Hb	93	g/L	115–165	g/L
HCT	0.266		0.37–0.47	
MCV	65.7	fL	80–100	fL
MCH	23.0	pg	26.5–33.0	pg
MCHC	350	g/L	310–360	g/L
RDW-SD	53.8	fL	38.0–48.0	fL
RDW-CV	15.9	%	12.0–14.5	%
RETIC CT				
RETIC ABS				
WBC	9.5	$\times 10^9/L$	3.5–11.0	$\times 10^9/L$
Plat	350	$\times 10^9/L$	150–400	$\times 10^9/L$

Differential						
Parameters	**Test Results**				**Reference Range**	
Neutrophil	76.7	%	7.2	$\times 10^9/L$	1.7–7.0	$\times 10^9/L$
Lymphocyte	20.3	%	1.9	$\times 10^9/L$	1.5–4.0	$\times 10^9/L$
Monocyte	2.0	%	0.2	$\times 10^9/L$	0.1–0.8	$\times 10^9/L$
Eosinophil	0.7	%	0.07	$\times 10^9/L$	0.04–0.44	$\times 10^9/L$
Basophil	0.3	%	0.03	$\times 10^9/L$	0.00–0.20	$\times 10^9/L$
NRBC	27 / 100 WBC					

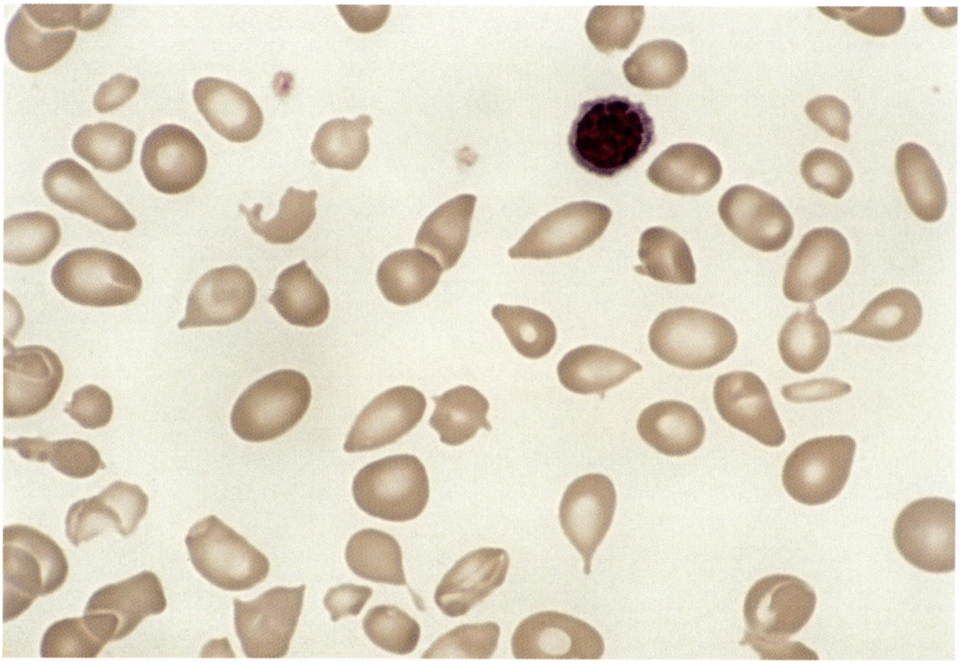

Blood film comments	
Red cell comments	Moderate anisocytosis Moderate microcytes Moderate hypochromasia Slight polychromasia Moderate teardrop poikilocytes 27 NRBC / 100 WBC
White cell comments	Neutrophilia
Platelet comments	Normal in number and morphology

Question 1. What is the differential diagnosis?

Based on the differential diagnosis, the following tests should be requested				
Haemoglobin electrophoresis (Hb EPG) Hb EPG cellulose acetate (pH 8.6)				
HbA_2	4.5	%	RR (2.0–3.5)	%
HbF	59.2	%	RR (<1)	%
Haemoglobin H inclusions not detected.				
Iron studies				
Iron	53.5	μmol/L	RR (8.1–32.6)	μmol/L
Transferrin	2.2	g/L	RR (1.8–3.3)	g/L
Iron saturation	97.3	%	RR (20–52)	%
Ferritin	2003	μg/L	RR (20–300)	μg/L

Question 2. Are further tests indicated as part of your final report? If so, which tests?

CASE STUDY 25

Case history

A 4-year-old child with severe anaemia for transfusion.

Analyser data

Parameters	Test Results		Reference Range	
RBC	3.14	× 10^{12}/L	3.96–4.92	× 10^{12}/L
Hb	76	g/L	110–139	g/L
HCT	0.238		0.32–0.39	
MCV	75.8	fL	74–86	fL
MCH	24.2	pg	25.5–30.6	pg
MCHC	319	g/L	310–360	g/L
RDW-SD	60.1	fL	34.3–44.1	fL
RDW-CV	20.1	%	12.1–15.6	%
RETIC CT	4.2	%	0.2–2.0	%
RETIC ABS	131.9	× 10^9/L	20–80	× 10^9/L
WBC	14.7	× 10^9/L	4.7–12.3	× 10^9/L
Plat	252	× 10^9/L	205–457	× 10^9/L

Differential

Parameters	Test Results				Reference Range	
Neutrophil	46.2	%	6.8	× 10^9/L	1.8–7.7	× 10^9/L
Lymphocyte	45.7	%	6.7	× 10^9/L	1.6–5.1	× 10^9/L
Monocyte	5.4	%	0.8	× 10^9/L	0.1–1.0	× 10^9/L
Eosinophil	2.4	%	0.36	× 10^9/L	0.00–0.60	× 10^9/L
Basophil NRBC	0.3 12 / 100 WBC	%	0.04	× 10^9/L	0.00–0.10	× 10^9/L

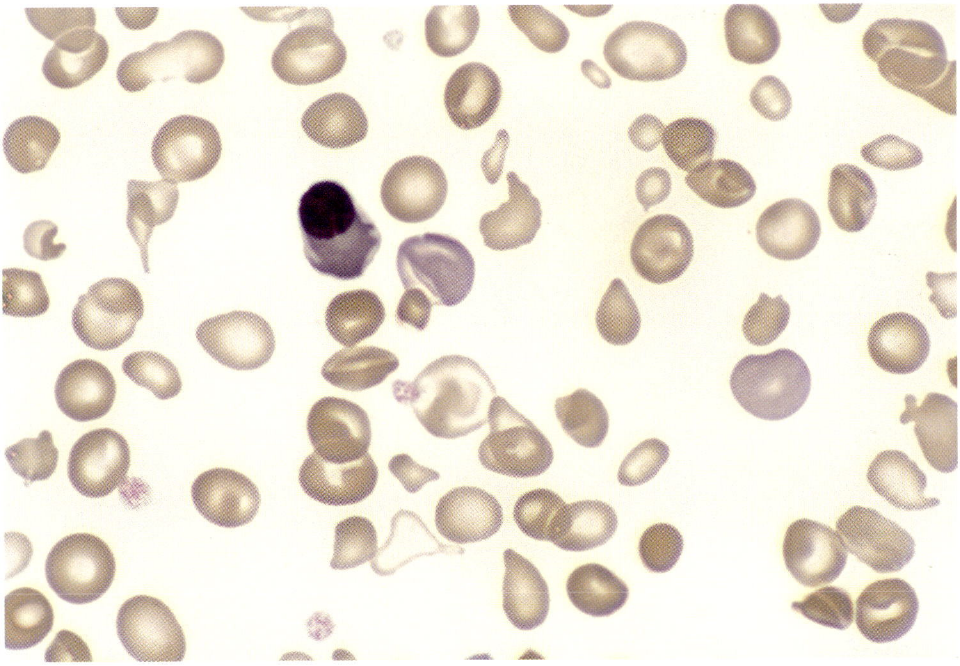

Blood film comments	
Red cell comments	Moderate anisocytosis Slight microcytes Slight hypochromasia Slight polychromasia 12 NRBC / 100 WBC
White cell comments	Lymphocytosis
Platelet comments	Normal in number and morphology

Question 1. What is the differential diagnosis?

Based on the differential diagnosis, the following tests should be requested				
Haemoglobin electrophoresis (Hb EPG) Hb EPG cellulose acetate (pH 8.6)				
HbA_2	1.0	%	RR (2.0–3.5)	%
HbF	95.9	%	RR (<1)	%
Haemoglobin H inclusions not detected.				
Iron studies				
Iron	26.7	μmol/L	RR (5.0–30.4)	μmol/L
Transferrin	1.0	g/L	RR (1.9–2.8)	g/L
Iron saturation	106.8	%	RR (16–51)	%
Ferritin	868	μg/L	RR (15–200)	μg/L

Question 2. Are further tests indicated as part of your final report? If so, which tests?

CASE STUDY 26

Case history

A 30-year-old female for antenatal blood count.

Analyser data				
Parameters	**Test Results**		**Reference Range**	
RBC	4.16	$\times 10^{12}/L$	3.80–5.80	$\times 10^{12}/L$
Hb	99	g/L	115–165	g/L
HCT	0.297		0.37–0.47	
MCV	73.1	fL	80–100	fL
MCH	23.8	pg	26.5–33.0	pg
MCHC	326	g/L	310–360	g/L
RDW-SD	46.5	fL	38.0–48.0	fL
RDW-CV	14.2	%	12.0–14.5	%
RETIC CT				
RETIC ABS				
WBC	12.5	$\times 10^9/L$	3.5–11.0	$\times 10^9/L$
Plat	354	$\times 10^9/L$	150–400	$\times 10^9/L$

Differential						
Parameters	**Test Results**				**Reference Range**	
Neutrophil	75.0	%	9.4	$\times 10^9/L$	1.7–7.0	$\times 10^9/L$
Lymphocyte	18.8	%	2.4	$\times 10^9/L$	1.5–4.0	$\times 10^9/L$
Monocyte	4.3	%	0.5	$\times 10^9/L$	0.1–0.8	$\times 10^9/L$
Eosinophil	1.7	%	0.21	$\times 10^9/L$	0.04–0.44	$\times 10^9/L$
Basophil	0.2	%	0.02	$\times 10^9/L$	0.00–0.20	$\times 10^9/L$

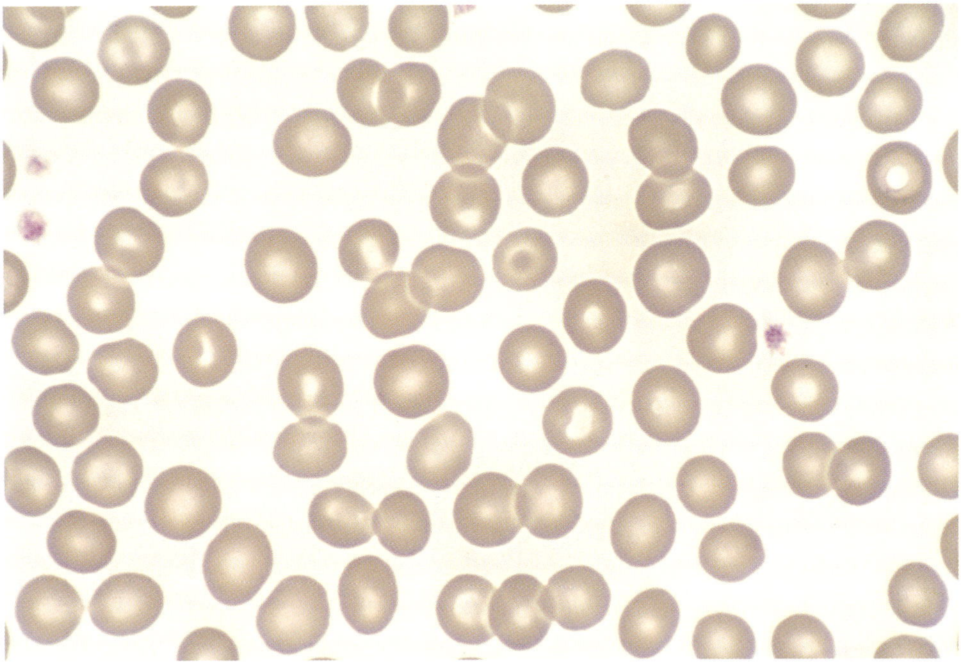

Blood film comments	
Red cell comments	Slight microcytes Slight hypochromasia Slight target cells
White cell comments	Neutrophilia
Platelet comments	Normal in number and morphology

Question 1. What is the differential diagnosis?

Based on the differential diagnosis, the following tests should be requested		
Haemoglobin electrophoresis (Hb EPG) Hb EPG cellulose acetate (pH 8.6)		
HbA_2 + HbE	28.9 %	
HbF	1.1 %	NR (<1) %
An abnormal band (HbE) is detected at the HbA_2 position. Haemoglobin H inclusions not detected. Iron studies are normal.		

Question 2. Are further tests indicated as part of your final report? If so, which tests?

CASE STUDY 27

Case history

A 3-year-old child from Southeast Asia having a blood count.

Analyser data

Parameters	Test Results		Reference Range	
RBC	6.55	$\times 10^{12}$/L	3.86–5.01	$\times 10^{12}$/L
Hb	121	g/L	107–136	g/L
HCT	0.363		0.31–0.38	
MCV	52.7	fL	73–85	fL
MCH	18.5	pg	24.8–29.9	pg
MCHC	351	g/L	310–360	g/L
RDW-SD	50.2	fL	34.3–44.1	fL
RDW-CV	15.9	%	12.1–15.6	%
RETIC CT				
RETIC ABS				
WBC	12.6	$\times 10^{9}$/L	4.9–12.8	$\times 10^{9}$/L
Plat	477	$\times 10^{9}$/L	214–483	$\times 10^{9}$/L

Differential

Parameters	Test Results				Reference Range	
Neutrophil	38.3	%	4.8	$\times 10^{9}$/L	1.7–6.7	$\times 10^{9}$/L
Lymphocyte	54.0	%	6.8	$\times 10^{9}$/L	2.0–6.6	$\times 10^{9}$/L
Monocyte	3.5	%	0.4	$\times 10^{9}$/L	0.2–1.0	$\times 10^{9}$/L
Eosinophil	3.7	%	0.47	$\times 10^{9}$/L	0.00–0.60	$\times 10^{9}$/L
Basophil	0.5	%	0.06	$\times 10^{9}$/L	0.00–0.10	$\times 10^{9}$/L

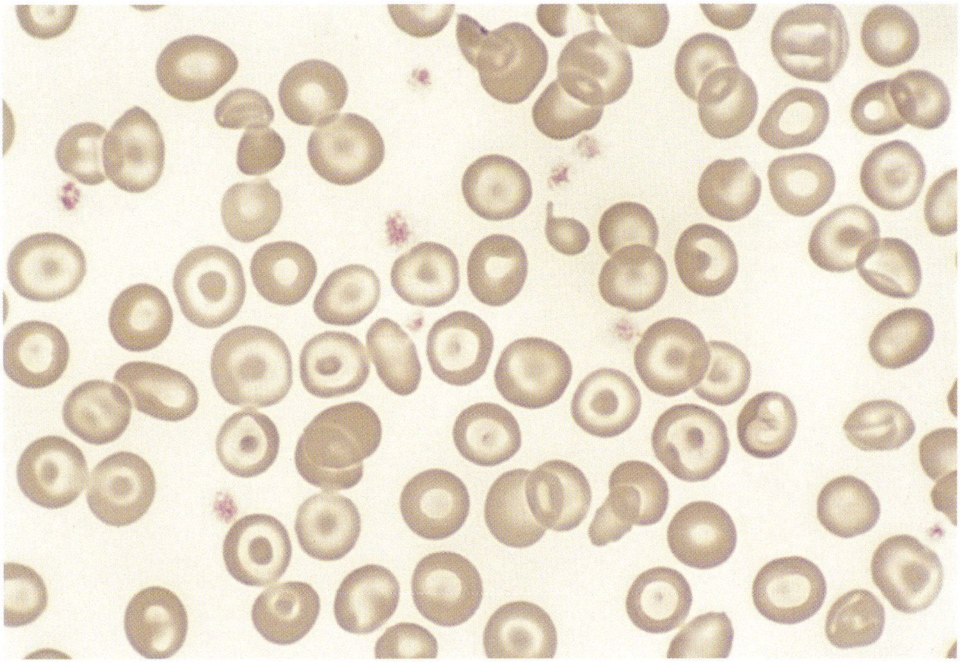

Blood film comments	
Red cell comments	Slight anisocytosis Slight microcytes Slight hypochromasia Marked target cells
White cell comments	Lymphocytosis
Platelet comments	Normal in number and morphology

Question 1. What is the differential diagnosis?

Based on the differential diagnosis, the following tests should be requested					
Haemoglobin electrophoresis (Hb EPG) Hb EPG cellulose acetate (pH 8.6)					
HbA_2 + HbE	84.5	%			
HbF	4.2	%	RR (<1)	%	
An abnormal band (HbE) is detected at the HbA_2 position. Haemoglobin H inclusions not detected. Iron studies are normal.					

Question 2. Are further tests indicated as part of your final report? If so, which tests?

CASE STUDY 28

Case history

A 47-year-old male from Ghana with severe bone pain.

Analyser data

Parameters	Test Results		Reference Range	
RBC	3.05	× 10^{12}/L	4.50–6.50	× 10^{12}/L
Hb	92	g/L	130–180	g/L
HCT	0.273		0.40–0.54	
MCV	89.5	fL	80–100	fL
MCH	30.2	pg	26.5–33.0	pg
MCHC	337	g/L	310–360	g/L
RDW-SD	49.7	fL	38.0–48.0	fL
RDW-CV	14.9	%	12.0–14.5	%
RETIC CT	3.9	%	0.2–2.0	%
RETIC ABS	119.0	× 10^9/L	20–80	× 10^9/L
WBC	13.2	× 10^9/L	3.5–11.0	× 10^9/L
Plat	217	× 10^9/L	150–400	× 10^9/L

Differential

Parameters	Test Results				Reference Range	
Neutrophil	61.5	%	8.1	× 10^9/L	1.7–7.0	× 10^9/L
Lymphocyte	23.8	%	3.1	× 10^9/L	1.5–4.0	× 10^9/L
Monocyte	9.7	%	1.3	× 10^9/L	0.1–0.8	× 10^9/L
Eosinophil	2.8	%	0.37	× 10^9/L	0.04–0.44	× 10^9/L
Basophil	2.2	%	0.29	× 10^9/L	0.00–0.20	× 10^9/L

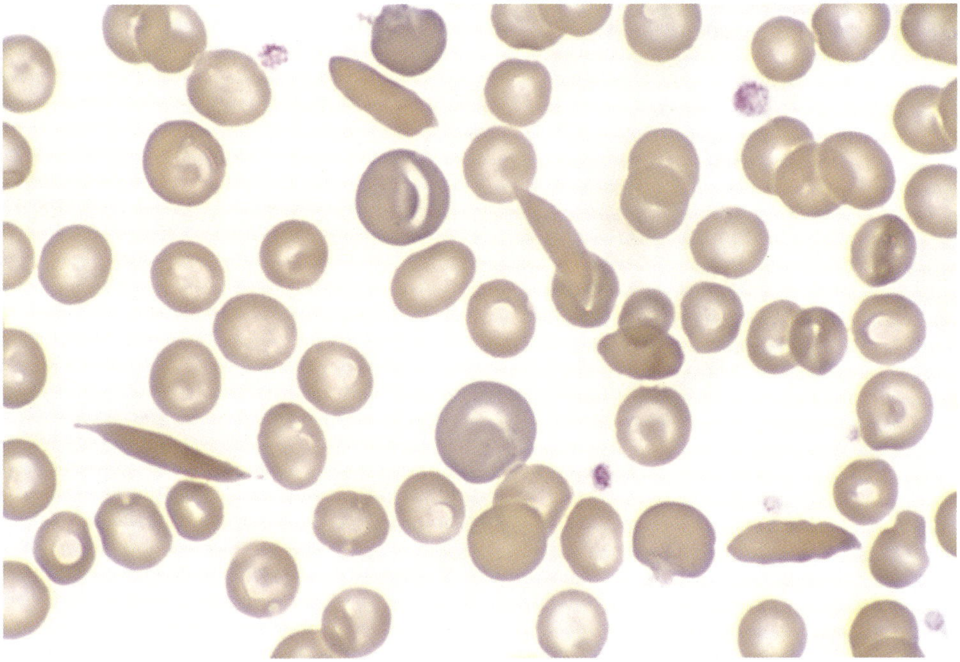

Blood film comments	
Red cell comments	Slight anisocytosis Slight polychromasia Slight target cells Moderate sickle cells
White cell comments	Neutrophilia
Platelet comments	Normal in number and morphology

Question 1. What is the differential diagnosis?

Based on the differential diagnosis, the following tests should be requested				
Haemoglobin electrophoresis (Hb EPG) Hb EPG cellulose acetate (pH 8.6): Abnormal band in HbS position. Hb EPG agar gel (pH 6.0): Abnormal band in HbS position.				
HbA_2	2.7	%	RR (2.0–3.5)	%
HbF	2.4	%	RR (<1)	%
HbS	28.6	%		
Haemoglobin H inclusions not detected.				
Ferritin	7145	μg/L	RR (20–300)	μg/L

Question 2. Are further tests indicated as part of your final report? If so, which tests?

CASE STUDY 29

Case history

A 20-year-old male from West Africa with splenomegaly and gall stones.

Analyser data				
Parameters	**Test Results**		**Reference Range**	
RBC	3.93	$\times 10^{12}$/L	4.50–6.50	$\times 10^{12}$/L
Hb	111	g/L	130–180	g/L
HCT	0.333		0.40–0.54	
MCV	78.9	fL	80–100	fL
MCH	27.2	pg	26.5–33.0	pg
MCHC	343	g/L	310–360	g/L
RDW-SD	48.7	fL	38.0–48.0	fL
RDW-CV	15.1	%	12.0–14.5	%
RETIC CT				
RETIC ABS				
WBC	7.5	$\times 10^9$/L	3.5–11.0	$\times 10^9$/L
Plat	204	$\times 10^9$/L	150–400	$\times 10^9$/L

Differential						
Parameters	**Test Results**				**Reference Range**	
Neutrophil	58.6	%	4.4	$\times 10^9$/L	1.7–7.0	$\times 10^9$/L
Lymphocyte	33.6	%	2.5	$\times 10^9$/L	1.5–4.0	$\times 10^9$/L
Monocyte	5.7	%	0.4	$\times 10^9$/L	0.1–0.8	$\times 10^9$/L
Eosinophil	1.3	%	0.10	$\times 10^9$/L	0.04–0.44	$\times 10^9$/L
Basophil	0.8	%	0.06	$\times 10^9$/L	0.00–0.20	$\times 10^9$/L

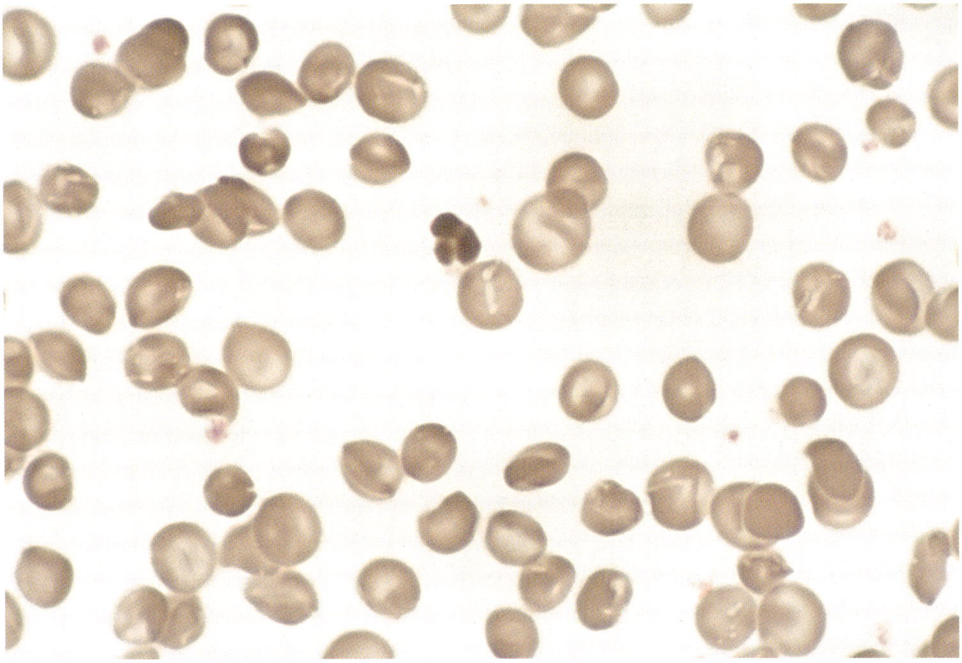

Blood film comments	
Red cell comments	Slight anisocytosis Slight microcytes Slight target cells Intraerythrocytic crystals of haemoglobin
White cell comments	Normal in number and morphology
Platelet comments	Normal in number and morphology

Question 1. What is the differential diagnosis?

Based on the differential diagnosis, the following tests should be requested				
Haemoglobin electrophoresis (Hb EPG) Hb EPG cellulose acetate (pH 8.6) Abnormal band (HbC) in the HbA_2 position. Hb EPG agar gel (pH 6.0): Abnormal band in the HbC position.				
HbA_2	3.2	%	RR (2.0–3.5)	%
HbF	0.8	%	RR (<1)	%
HbC	96.0	%		
Iron studies are normal.				

Question 2. Are further tests indicated as part of your final report? If so, which tests?

CASE STUDY 30

Case history

An 8-year-old child with third degree burns to 75% of the body.

Analyser data				
Parameters	**Test Results**		**Reference Range**	
RBC	6.43	$\times 10^{12}/L$	3.96–4.92	$\times 10^{12}/L$
Hb	118	g/L	110–139	g/L
HCT	0.349		0.32–0.39	
MCV	53.3	fL	74–86	fL
MCH	18.4	pg	25.5–30.6	pg
MCHC	344	g/L	310–360	g/L
RDW-SD	74.0	fL	35.3–41.0	fL
RDW-CV	15.7	%	12.0–14.1	%
RETIC CT				
RETIC ABS				
WBC	34.3	$\times 10^9/L$	4.7–12.3	$\times 10^9/L$
Plat	No result due to the presence of red cell fragmentation		187–415	$\times 10^9/L$

Differential						
Parameters	**Test Results**				**Reference Range**	
Neutrophil	57.0	%	19.5	$\times 10^9/L$	1.8–7.7	$\times 10^9/L$
Lymphocyte	37.0	%	12.7	$\times 10^9/L$	1.6–5.1	$\times 10^9/L$
Monocyte	2.3	%	0.8	$\times 10^9/L$	0.1–1.0	$\times 10^9/L$
Eosinophil	3.3	%	1.14	$\times 10^9/L$	0.00–0.60	$\times 10^9/L$
Basophil	0.4	%	0.15	$\times 10^9/L$	0.00–0.10	$\times 10^9/L$

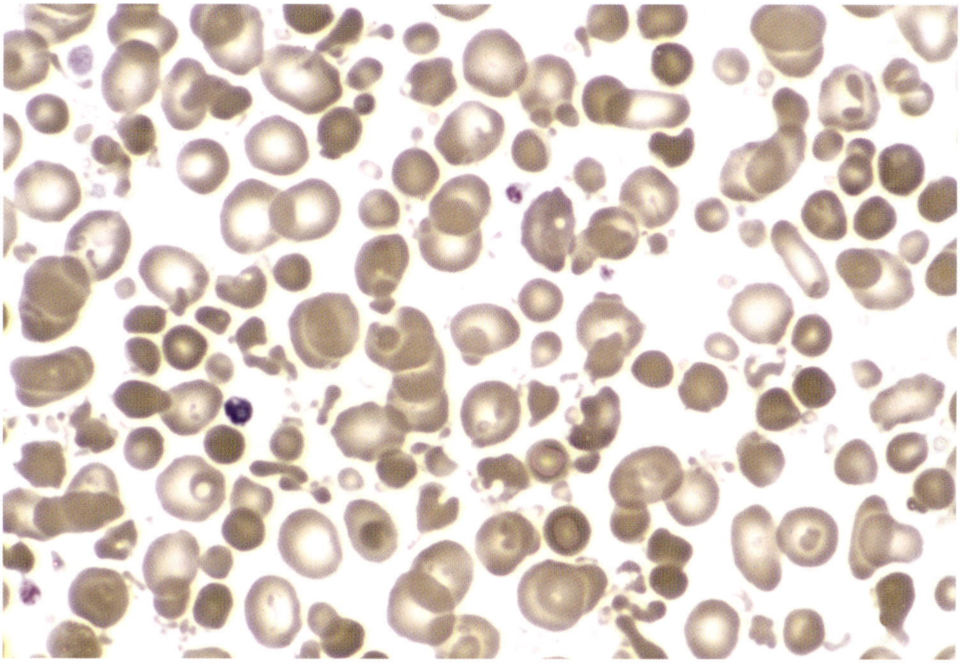

Blood film comments	
Red cell comments	Marked anisocytosis Moderate microcytes Moderate hypochromasia Marked fragments Marked microspherocytes Marked red cell budding
White cell comments	Neutrophilia
Platelet comments	False high platelet count due to the presence of red cell fragmentation – no result issued.

Question 1. What is the differential diagnosis?

Based on the differential diagnosis, the following tests should be requested
The red cell count, MCV and MCH are suggestive of thalassaemia trait; however no further testing was performed.

Question 2. Are further tests indicated as part of your final report? If so, which tests?

CASE STUDY 31

Case history

A 37-year-old female preoperative blood test.

Analyser data				
Parameters	**Test Results**		**Reference Range**	
RBC	4.23	$\times 10^{12}/L$	3.80–5.80	$\times 10^{12}/L$
Hb	125	g/L	115–165	g/L
HCT	0.375		0.37–0.47	
MCV	86.3	fL	80–100	
MCH	29.6	pg	26.5–33.0	pg
MCHC	342	g/L	310–360	g/L
RDW-SD	38.7	fL	38.0–48.0	fL
RDW-CV	14.5	%	12.0–14.5	%
RETIC CT				
RETIC ABS				
WBC	11.0	$\times 10^9/L$	3.5–11.0	$\times 10^9/L$
Plat	204	$\times 10^9/L$	150–400	$\times 10^9/L$

Differential						
Parameters	**Test Results**				**Reference Range**	
Neutrophil	79.6	%	8.8	$\times 10^9/L$	1.7–7.0	$\times 10^9/L$
Lymphocyte	12.5	%	1.4	$\times 10^9/L$	1.5–4.0	$\times 10^9/L$
Monocyte	5.6	%	0.6	$\times 10^9/L$	0.1–0.8	$\times 10^9/L$
Eosinophil	1.8	%	0.20	$\times 10^9/L$	0.04–0.44	$\times 10^9/L$
Basophil	0.5	%	0.05	$\times 10^9/L$	0.00–0.20	$\times 10^9/L$

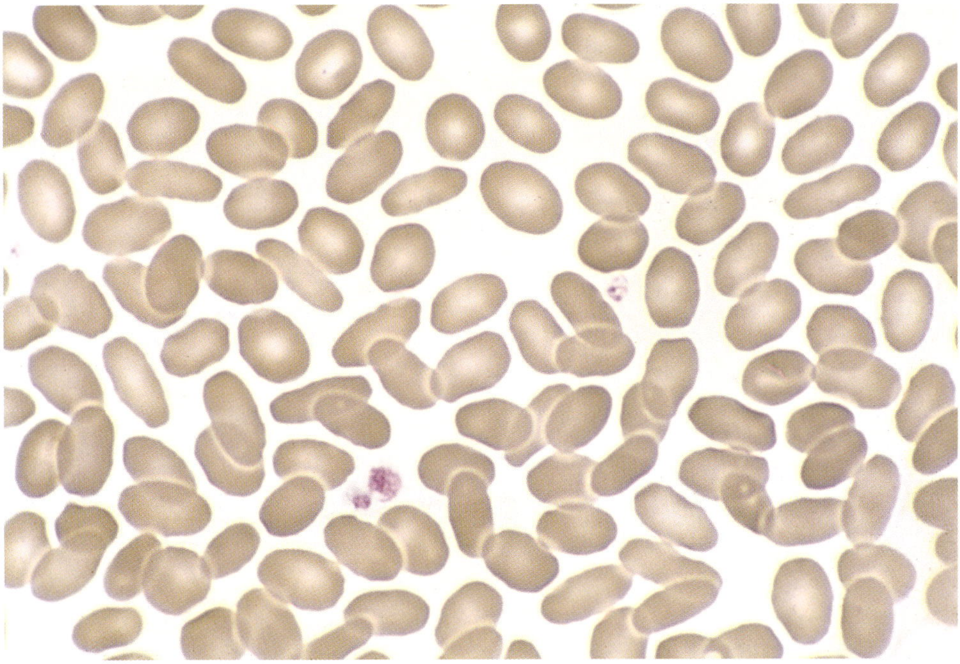

Blood film comments	
Red cell comments	Marked elliptocytes
White cell comments	Neutrophilia
Platelet comments	Normal in number and morphology

Question 1. What is the differential diagnosis?

Based on the differential diagnosis, the following tests should be requested
No further tests are indicated. The image is diagnostic of hereditary elliptocytosis.

Question 2. Are further tests required as part of your final report? If so, which tests?

CASE STUDY 32

Case history

A 54-year-old male postoperative craniotomy.

Analyser data				
Parameters	**Test Results**		**Reference Range**	
RBC	4.51	$\times 10^{12}/L$	4.50–6.50	$\times 10^{12}/L$
Hb	140	g/L	130–180	g/L
HCT	0.420		0.40–0.54	
MCV	86.3	fL	80–100	fL
MCH	31.0	pg	26.5–33.0	pg
MCHC	355	g/L	310–360	g/L
RDW-SD	47.1	fL	38.0–48.0	fL
RDW-CV	14.2	%	12.0–14.5	%
RETIC CT				
RETIC ABS				
WBC	18.4	$\times 10^9/L$	3.5–11.0	$\times 10^9/L$
Plat	165	$\times 10^9/L$	150–400	$\times 10^9/L$

Differential						
Parameters	**Test Results**				**Reference Range**	
Neutrophil	89.8	%	16.6	$\times 10^9/L$	1.7–7.0	$\times 10^9/L$
Lymphocyte	5.5	%	1.0	$\times 10^9/L$	1.5–4.0	$\times 10^9/L$
Monocyte	4.7	%	0.8	$\times 10^9/L$	0.1–0.8	$\times 10^9/L$
Eosinophil	0.0	%	0.00	$\times 10^9/L$	0.04–0.44	$\times 10^9/L$
Basophil	0.0	%	0.00	$\times 10^9/L$	0.00–0.20	$\times 10^9/L$

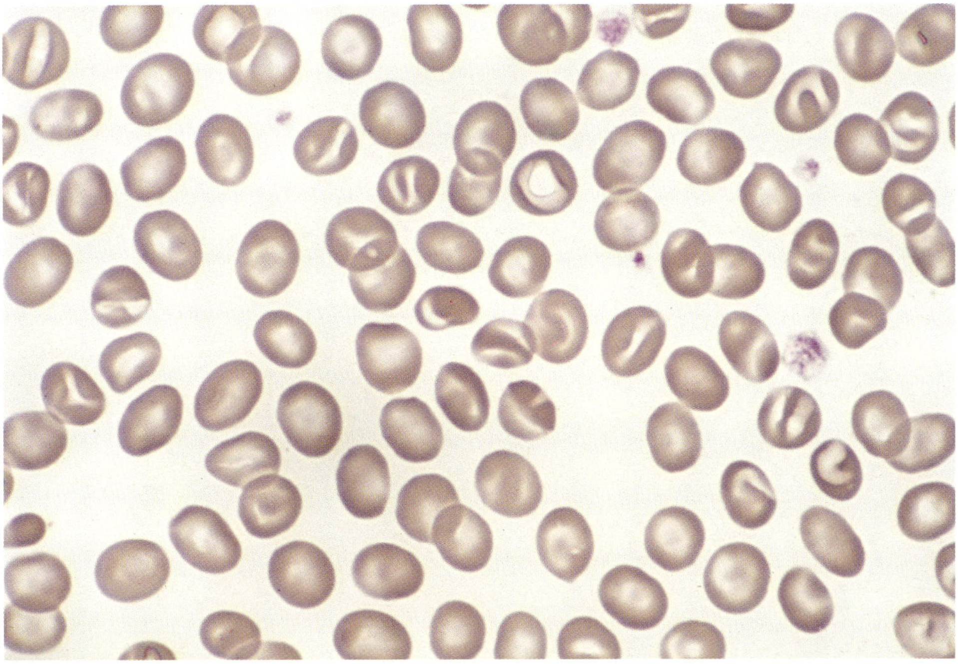

Blood film comments	
Red cell comments	Marked ovalocytes Marked stomatocytes
White cell comments	Neutrophilia
Platelet comments	Normal in number and morphology

Question 1. What is the differential diagnosis?

Based on the differential diagnosis, the following tests should be requested
No further tests are indicated. The image is diagnostic of Southeast Asian ovalocytosis.

Question 2. Are further tests indicated as part of your final report? If so, which tests?

CASE STUDY 33

Case history

A 27-year-old male with a history of anaemia having a checkup blood count.

Analyser data				
Parameters	**Test Results**		**Reference Range**	
RBC	4.62	$\times 10^{12}$/L	4.50–6.50	$\times 10^{12}$/L
Hb	105	g/L	130–180	g/L
HCT	0.315		0.40–0.54	
MCV	130.2	fL	80–100	fL
MCH	48.7	pg	26.5–33.0	pg
MCHC	315	g/L	310–360	g/L
RDW-SD	57.0	fL	38.0–48.0	fL
RDW-CV	16.2	%	12.0–14.5	%
RETIC CT	3.9	%	0.2–2.0	%
RETIC ABS	180.2	$\times 10^9$/L	20–80	$\times 10^9$/L
WBC	12.0	$\times 10^9$/L	3.5–11.0	$\times 10^9$/L
Plat	353	$\times 10^9$/L	150–400	$\times 10^9$/L

Differential						
Parameters	**Test Results**				**Reference Range**	
Neutrophil	61.8	%	7.4	$\times 10^9$/L	1.7–7.0	$\times 10^9$/L
Lymphocyte	28.5	%	3.4	$\times 10^9$/L	1.5–4.0	$\times 10^9$/L
Monocyte	6.1	%	0.7	$\times 10^9$/L	0.1–0.8	$\times 10^9$/L
Eosinophil	2.9	%	0.35	$\times 10^9$/L	0.04–0.44	$\times 10^9$/L
Basophil	0.7	%	0.08	$\times 10^9$/L	0.00–0.20	$\times 10^9$/L

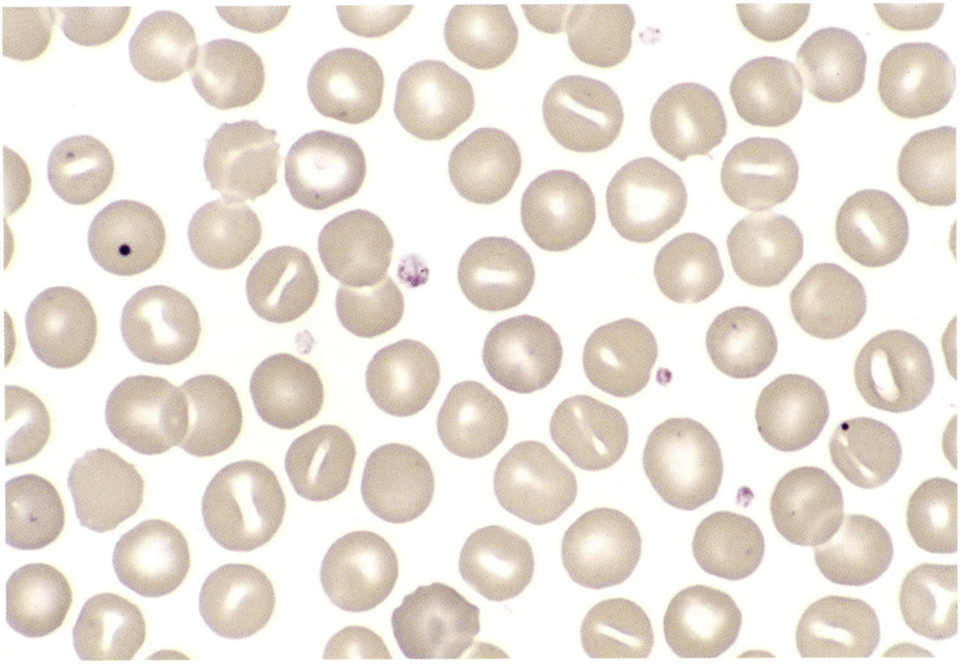

Blood film comments	
Red cell comments	Slight anisocytosis Marked macrocytes Slight polychromasia Moderate stomatocytes Slight Pappenheimer bodies Occasional Howell Jolly body
White cell comments	Neutrophilia
Platelet comments	Normal in number and morphology

Question 1. What is the differential diagnosis?

Based on the differential diagnosis, the following tests should be requested
The image together with the significantly raised MCV are suggestive of hereditary stomatocytosis.

Question 2. Are further tests indicated as part of your final report? If so, which tests?

CASE STUDY 34

Case history

A 5-month-old child with 'failure to thrive'.

Analyser data				
Parameters	**Test Results**		**Reference Range**	
RBC	5.05	× 10^{12}/L	3.39–4.86	× 10^{12}/L
Hb	150	g/L	100–122	g/L
HCT	0.453		0.28–0.36	
MCV	84.2	fL	68–85	fL
MCH	29.7	pg	22.6–29.7	pg
MCHC	353	g/L	310–360	g/L
RDW-SD	43.1	fL	34.0–42.4	fL
RDW-CV	13.8	%	12.0–14.8	%
RETIC CT				
RETIC ABS				
WBC	8.2	× 10^9/L	5.6–14.1	× 10^9/L
Plat	433	× 10^9/L	295–685	× 10^9/L

Differential						
Parameters	**Test Results**				**Reference Range**	
Neutrophil	20.0	%	1.6	× 10^9/L	0.5–4.4	× 10^9/L
Lymphocyte	74.0	%	6.1	× 10^9/L	3.4–9.8	× 10^9/L
Monocyte	6.0	%	0.5	× 10^9/L	0.2–1.0	× 10^9/L
Eosinophil	0.0	%	0.00	× 10^9/L	0.00–0.7	× 10^9/L
Basophil	0.0	%	0.00	× 10^9/L	0.00–0.10	× 10^9/L

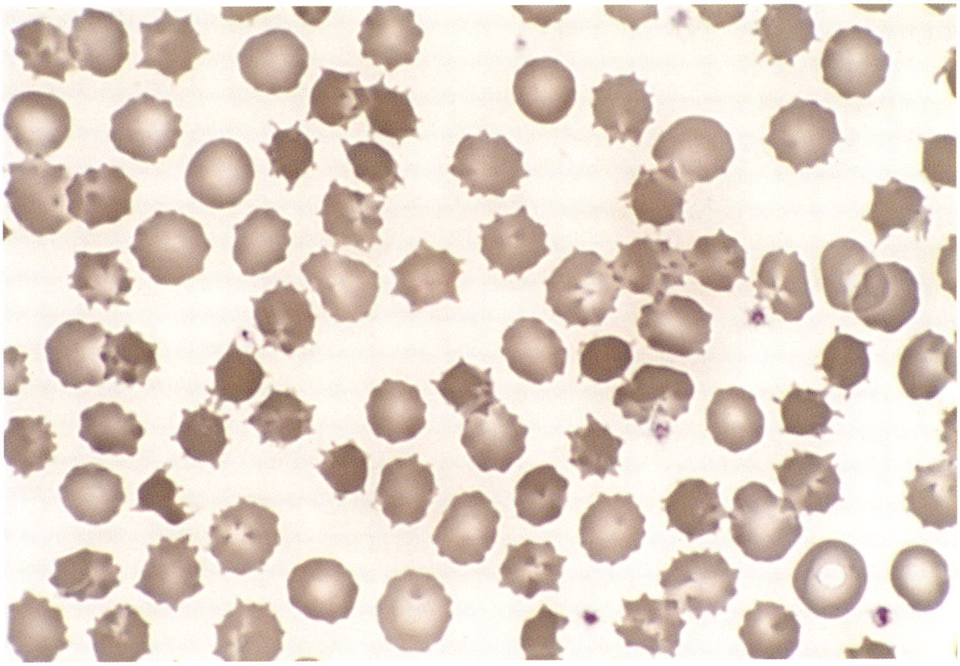

Blood film comments	
Red cell comments	Slight anisocytosis Marked acanthocytes
White cell comments	Normal in number and morphology
Platelet comments	Normal in number and morphology

Question 1. What is the differential diagnosis?

Based on the differential diagnosis, the following tests should be requested				
Cholesterol	1.4	mmol/L	RR (3.0–5.5)	mmol/L
Triglyceride	<0.1	mmol/L	RR (<2.0)	mmol/L
HDL	1.3	mmol/L	RR (0.9–2.4)	mmol/L
Vitamin E	<1	μmol/L	RR (5–14)	μmol/L

Question 2. Are further tests indicated as part of your final report? If so, which tests?

CASE STUDY 35

Case history

A 64-year-old female with chronic anaemia.

Analyser data				
Parameters	**Test Results**		**Reference Range**	
RBC	2.78	× 10^{12}/L	3.80–5.80	× 10^{12}/L
Hb	80	g/L	115–165	g/L
HCT	0.246		0.37–0.47	
MCV	92.1	fL	80–100	fL
MCH	28.8	pg	26.5–33.0	pg
MCHC	313	g/L	310–360	g/L
RDW-SD	55.3	fL	38.0–48.0	fL
RDW-CV	16.8	%	12.0–14.5	%
RETIC CT				
RETIC ABS				
WBC	13.6	× 10^9/L	3.5–11.0	× 10^9/L
Plat	416	× 10^9/L	150–400	× 10^9/L
ESR	68 mm/h		<20 mm/h	

Differential						
Parameters	**Test Results**				**Reference Range**	
Neutrophil	79.4	%	10.8	× 10^9/L	1.7–7.0	× 10^9/L
Lymphocyte	6.6	%	0.9	× 10^9/L	1.5–4.0	× 10^9/L
Monocyte	3.5	%	0.5	× 10^9/L	0.1–0.8	× 10^9/L
Eosinophil	9.7	%	1.33	× 10^9/L	0.04–0.44	× 10^9/L
Basophil	0.8	%	0.11	× 10^9/L	0.00–0.20	× 10^9/L

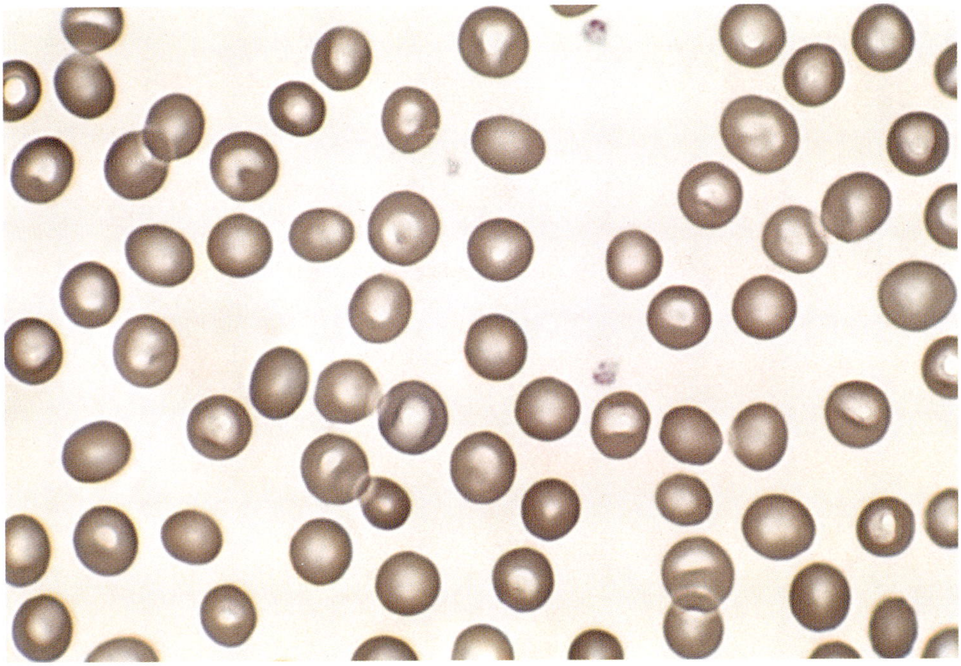

Blood film comments	
Red cell comments	Slight anisocytosis Slight rouleaux
White cell comments	Neutrophilia Eosinophilia
Platelet comments	Thrombocytosis

Question 1. What is the differential diagnosis?

Based on the differential diagnosis, the following tests should be requested				
Urea	21.0	mmol/L	RR (2.9–7.1)	mmol/L
Creatinine	660	μmol/L	RR (60–110)	μmol/L

Question 2. Are further tests indicated as part of your final report? If so, which tests?

CASE STUDY 36

Case history

A 95-year-old female febrile and anuric.

Analyser data				
Parameters	**Test Results**		**Reference Range**	
RBC	3.81	$\times 10^{12}$/L	3.80–5.80	$\times 10^{12}$/L
Hb	118	g/L	115–165	g/L
HCT	0.354		0.37–0.47	
MCV	92.1	fL	80–100	fL
MCH	31.0	pg	26.5–33.0	
MCHC	336	g/L	310–360	g/L
RDW-SD	53.3	fL	38.0–48.0	fL
RDW-CV	15.9	%	12.0–14.5	%
RETIC CT				
RETIC ABS				
WBC	17.8	$\times 10^9$/L	3.5–11.0	$\times 10^9$/L
Plat	138	$\times 10^9$/L	150–400	$\times 10^9$/L

Differential						
Parameters	**Test Results**				**Reference Range**	
Neutrophil	93.3	%	16.7	$\times 10^9$/L	1.7–7.0	$\times 10^9$/L
Lymphocyte	2.9	%	0.5	$\times 10^9$/L	1.5–4.0	$\times 10^9$/L
Monocyte	3.1	%	0.6	$\times 10^9$/L	0.1–0.8	$\times 10^9$/L
Eosinophil	0.0	%	0.00	$\times 10^9$/L	0.04–0.44	$\times 10^9$/L
Basophil	0.1	%	0.01	$\times 10^9$/L	0.00–0.20	$\times 10^9$/L

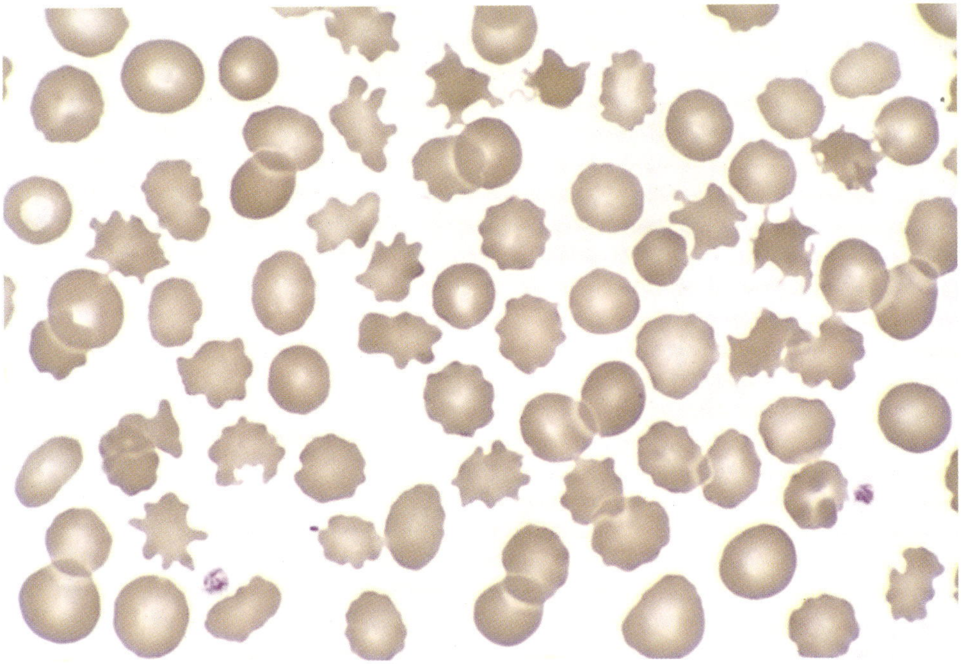

Blood film comments	
Red cell comments	Slight anisocytosis Moderate burr cells Slight rouleaux
White cell comments	Neutrophilia
Platelet comments	Thrombocytopenia

Question 1. What is the differential diagnosis?

Based on the differential diagnosis, the following tests should be requested				
Urea	66.1	mmol/L	RR (2.9–7.1)	mmol/L
Creatinine	904	μmol/L	RR (60–110)	μmol/L

Question 2. Are further tests indicated as part of your final report? If so, which tests?

CASE STUDY 37

Case history

A 71-year-old male post multiple trauma.

Analyser data				
Parameters	**Test Results**		**Reference Range**	
RBC	3.97	× 10^{12}/L	4.50–6.50	× 10^{12}/L
Hb	116	g/L	130–180	g/L
HCT	0.348		0.40–0.54	
MCV	90.4	fL	80–100	fL
MCH	29.2	pg	26.5–33.0	pg
MCHC	323	g/L	310–360	g/L
RDW-SD	50.2	fL	38.0–48.0	fL
RDW-CV	15.3	%	12.0–14.5	%
RETIC CT				
RETIC ABS				
WBC	9.6	× 10^9/L	3.5–11.0	× 10^9/L
Plat	1072	× 10^9/L	150–400	× 10^9/L

Differential						
Parameters	**Test Results**				**Reference Range**	
Neutrophil	68.3	%	6.6	× 10^9/L	1.7–7.0	× 10^9/L
Lymphocyte	22.8	%	2.2	× 10^9/L	1.5–4.0	× 10^9/L
Monocyte	5.5	%	0.5	× 10^9/L	0.1–0.8	× 10^9/L
Eosinophil	3.1	%	0.30	× 10^9/L	0.04–0.44	× 10^9/L
Basophil	0.3	%	0.03	× 10^9/L	0.00–0.20	× 10^9/L

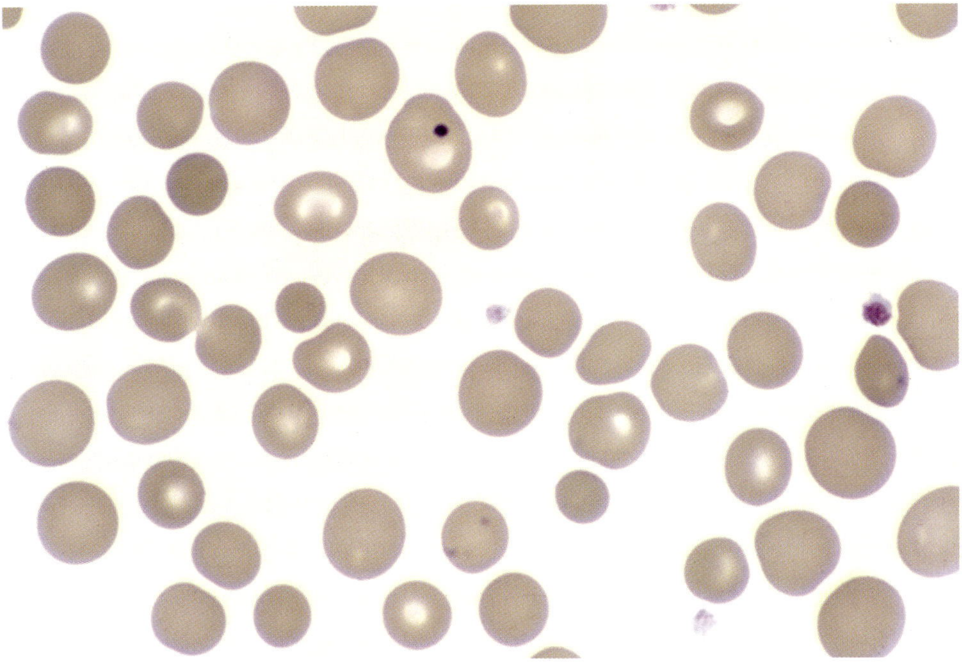

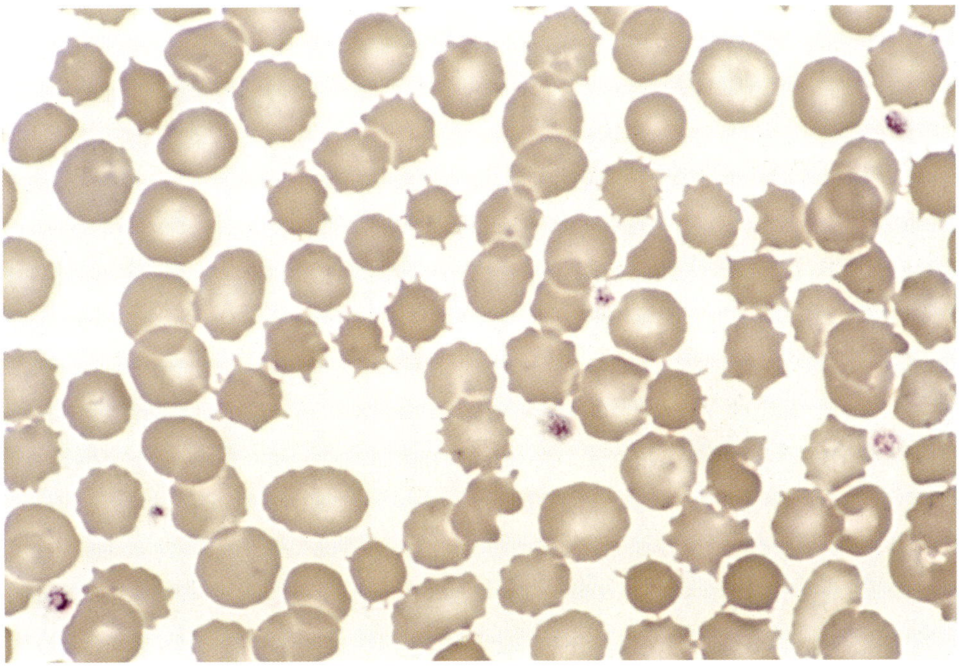

Blood film comments	
Red cell comments	Slight anisocytosis Slight target cells Slight acanthocytes Slight Howell Jolly bodies
White cell comments	Normal in number and morphology
Platelet comments	Thrombocytosis

Question 1. What is the differential diagnosis?

Based on the differential diagnosis, the following tests should be requested
Diagnostic blood film. No further tests are indicated.

Question 2. Are further tests indicated as part of your final report? If so, which tests?

3
White Cell Cases

CASE STUDY 38

Case history

A 64-year-old male presents with lassitude, anaemia and splenomegaly.

Analyser data				
Parameters	**Test Results**		**Reference Range**	
RBC	3.64	$\times 10^{12}$/L	4.50–6.50	$\times 10^{12}$/L
Hb	104	g/L	130–180	g/L
HCT	0.316		0.40–0.54	
MCV	86.8	fL	80–100	fL
MCH	28.6	pg	26.5–33.0	pg
MCHC	329	g/L	310–360	g/L
RDW-SD	48.7	fL	38.0–48.0	fL
RDW-CV	15.2	%	12.0–14.5	%
RETIC CT				
RETIC ABS				
WBC	170.6	$\times 10^9$/L	3.5–11.0	$\times 10^9$/L
Plat	338	$\times 10^9$/L	150–400	$\times 10^9$/L

Differential						
Parameters	**Test Results**				**Reference Range**	
Neutrophil	45.0	%	76.8	$\times 10^9$/L	1.7–7.0	$\times 10^9$/L
Lymphocyte	2.0	%	3.4	$\times 10^9$/L	1.5–4.0	$\times 10^9$/L
Monocyte	3.0	%	5.1	$\times 10^9$/L	0.1–0.8	$\times 10^9$/L
Eosinophil	3.0	%	5.1	$\times 10^9$/L	0.04–0.44	$\times 10^9$/L
Basophil	8.0	%	13.6	$\times 10^9$/L	0.00–0.20	$\times 10^9$/L
Blast	3	%				
Promyelocyte	2	%				
Metamyelocyte	4	%				
Myelocyte	21	%				
Band form	9	%				
NRBC	3 / 100 WBC					

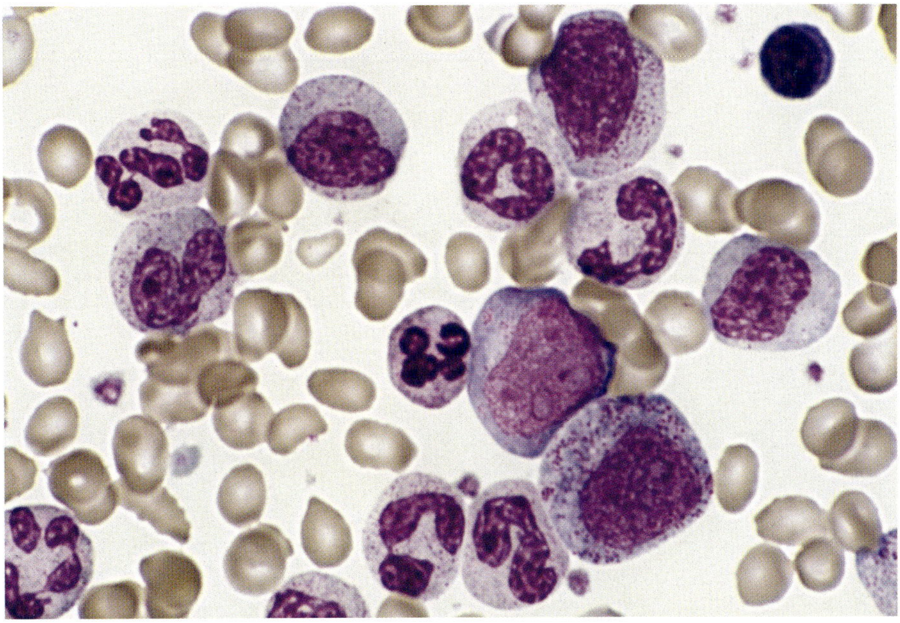

Blood film comments	
Red cell comments	Slight anisocytosis 3 NRBC / 100 WBC
White blood cell comments	Left shift in the myeloid line Neutrophilia Eosinophilia Basophilia 3% blasts Leucoerythroblastic blood picture
Platelet comments	Normal in number and morphology

Question 1. What is the differential diagnosis?

Based on the differential diagnosis, the following tests should be requested	
Bone marrow, trephine and cytogenetics	
Bone marrow	Markedly hypercellular marrow with myeloid proliferation, consistent with chronic myelogenous leukaemia, likely chronic phase.
Trephine	Bone marrow trephine as above.
Cytogenetics	Chromosome analysis revealed an abnormal clone t(9;22)(q34;q11.2). No normal cells were seen. All cells contained a translocation between the long arms of chromosomes 9 and 22. FISH confirmed the fusion of the *BCR/ABL* genes and no cryptic deletion of the derivative 9 chromosome was found.

Question 2. Are further tests indicated as part of your final report? If so, which tests?

CASE STUDY 39

Case history

A 70-year-old male with a history of headaches, pruritus and gastrointestinal bleeding.

Analyser data				
Parameters	**Test Results**		**Reference Range**	
RBC	7.46	$\times 10^{12}/L$	4.50–6.50	$\times 10^{12}/L$
Hb	189	g/L	130–180	g/L
HCT	0.600		0.40–0.54	
MCV	80.4	fL	80–100	fL
MCH	25.3	pg	26.5–33.0	pg
MCHC	315	g/L	310–360	g/L
RDW-SD	49.2	fL	38.0–48.0	fL
RDW-CV	15.9	%	12.0–14.5	%
RETIC CT				
RETIC ABS				
WBC	15.1	$\times 10^9/L$	3.5–11.0	$\times 10^9/L$
Plat	428	$\times 10^9/L$	150–400	$\times 10^9/L$

Differential						
Parameters	**Test Results**				**Reference Range**	
Neutrophil	80.9	%	12.2	$\times 10^9/L$	1.7–7.0	$\times 10^9/L$
Lymphocyte	12.2	%	1.9	$\times 10^9/L$	1.5–4.0	$\times 10^9/L$
Monocyte	2.4	%	0.4	$\times 10^9/L$	0.1–0.8	$\times 10^9/L$
Eosinophil	2.6	%	0.40	$\times 10^9/L$	0.04–0.44	$\times 10^9/L$
Basophil	1.9	%	0.29	$\times 10^9/L$	0.00–0.20	$\times 10^9/L$

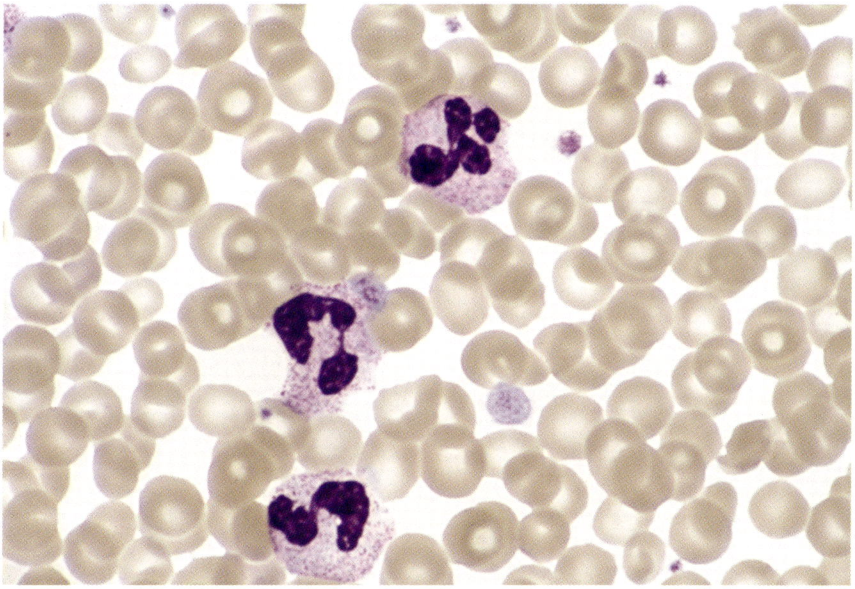

Blood film comments	
Red cell comments	Slight anisocytosis Slight microcytes Slight hypochromasia Note raised Hb. ? dehydration ? polycythaemia
White blood cell comments	Neutrophilia Basophilia
Platelet comments	Thrombocytosis Large and giant platelets present

Question 1. What is the differential diagnosis?

Based on the differential diagnosis, the following tests should be requested
Bone marrow and trephine studies no longer tend to be performed when making a diagnosis of polycythaemia vera.
Molecular genetics *JAK2* V617F: Positive.
More than 95 % of patients with polycythaemia vera carry the gain-of-function mutation Janus 2 kinase gene, *JAK2* V617F; however, these mutations are not specific for polycythaemia vera. A functionally similar mutation in exon 12 of *JAK2* may also be present.

Question 2. Are further tests indicated as part of your final report? If so, which tests?

Iron studies				
Iron	5.7	µmol/L	RR (8.1–32.6)	µmol/L
Transferrin	4.2	g/L	RR (1.8–3.3)	g/L
Iron saturation	6.6	%	RR (20–52)	%
Ferritin	12	µg/L	RR (20–300)	µg/L

CASE STUDY 40

Case history

A 63-year-old female with weakness, shortness of breath on exertion and enlarged spleen.

Analyser data				
Parameters	**Test Results**		**Reference Range**	
RBC	3.74	$\times 10^{12}/L$	3.80–5.80	$\times 10^{12}/L$
Hb	91	g/L	115–165	g/L
HCT	0.312		0.37–0.47	
MCV	83.4	fL	80–100	fL
MCH	24.3	pg	26.5–33.0	pg
MCHC	292	g/L	310–360	g/L
RDW-SD	51.6	fL	38.0–48.0	fL
RDW-CV	16.2	%	12.0–14.5	%
RETIC CT				
RETIC ABS				
WBC	14.6	$\times 10^9/L$	3.5–11.0	$\times 10^9/L$
Plat	530	$\times 10^9/L$	150–400	$\times 10^9/L$

Differential						
Parameters	**Test Results**				**Reference Range**	
Neutrophil	72.0	%	10.5	$\times 10^9/L$	1.7–7.0	$\times 10^9/L$
Lymphocyte	4.0	%	0.6	$\times 10^9/L$	1.5–4.0	$\times 10^9/L$
Monocyte	6.0	%	0.9	$\times 10^9/L$	0.1–0.8	$\times 10^9/L$
Eosinophil	2.0	%	0.29	$\times 10^9/L$	0.04–0.44	$\times 10^9/L$
Basophil	3.0	%	0.44	$\times 10^9/L$	0.00–0.20	$\times 10^9/L$
Blast	3	%				
Metamyelocyte	1	%				
NRBC	1 / 100 WBC					

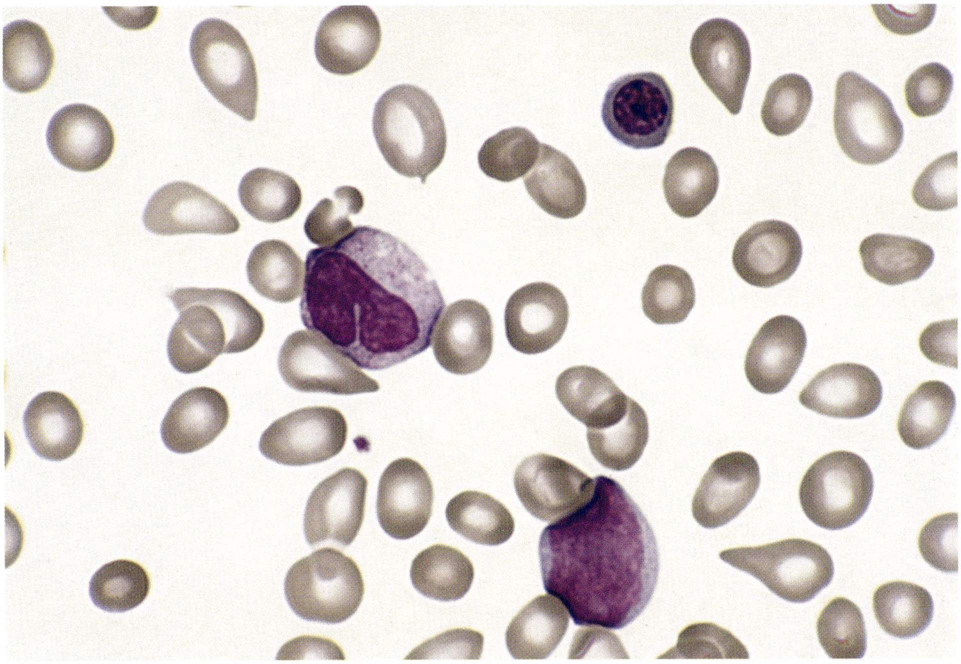

Blood film comments	
Red cell comments	Slight anisocytosis Slight microcytes Slight hypochromasia Slight teardrop poikilocytes 1 NRBC / 100 WBC
White blood cell comments	Left shift in the myeloid line Neutrophilia Basophilia 3 % blasts Leucoerythroblastic blood film
Platelet comments	Thrombocytosis Large platelets present

Question 1. What is the differential diagnosis?

Based on the differential diagnosis, the following tests should be requested	
Bone marrow, trephine and cytogenetics	
Bone marrow	Dry tap.
Trephine	Myeloid hyperplasia and increased megakaryopoiesis. The megakaryocytes are multinucleated and forming clusters. There is markedly increased fibrosis which is confirmed by performing a reticulum stain.

Molecular genetics	*JAK2* V617F: Positive. Approximately 50% of patients with primary myelofibrosis carry the *JAK2* V617F mutation gene.
Iron studies may be indicated.	

Question 2. Are further tests indicated as part of your final report? If so, which tests?

CASE STUDY 41

Case history

A 62-year-old female with a mild splenomegaly who is otherwise well.

Analyser data				
Parameters	**Test Results**		**Reference Range**	
RBC	5.90	$\times 10^{12}$/L	3.80–5.80	$\times 10^{12}$/L
Hb	139	g/L	115–165	g/L
HCT	0.461		0.37–0.47	
MCV	78.1	fL	80–100	fL
MCH	23.6	pg	26.5–33.0	pg
MCHC	302	g/L	310–360	g/L
RDW-SD	49.3	fL	38.0–48.0	fL
RDW-CV	17.9	%	12.0–14.5	%
RETIC CT				
RETIC ABS				
WBC	10.3	$\times 10^9$/L	3.5–11.0	$\times 10^9$/L
Plat	908	$\times 10^9$/L	150–400	$\times 10^9$/L

Differential						
Parameters	**Test Results**				**Reference Range**	
Neutrophil	87.8	%	9.0	$\times 10^9$/L	1.7–7.0	$\times 10^9$/L
Lymphocyte	8.3	%	0.9	$\times 10^9$/L	1.5–4.0	$\times 10^9$/L
Monocyte	1.7	%	0.2	$\times 10^9$/L	0.1–0.8	$\times 10^9$/L
Eosinophil	1.6	%	0.16	$\times 10^9$/L	0.04–0.44	$\times 10^9$/L
Basophil	0.6	%	0.06	$\times 10^9$/L	0.00–0.20	$\times 10^9$/L

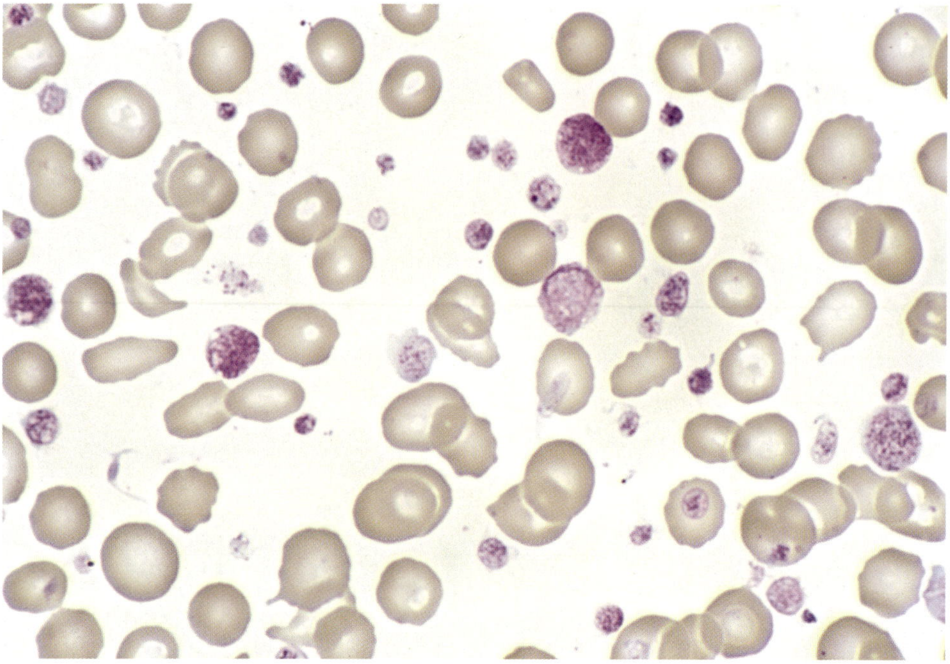

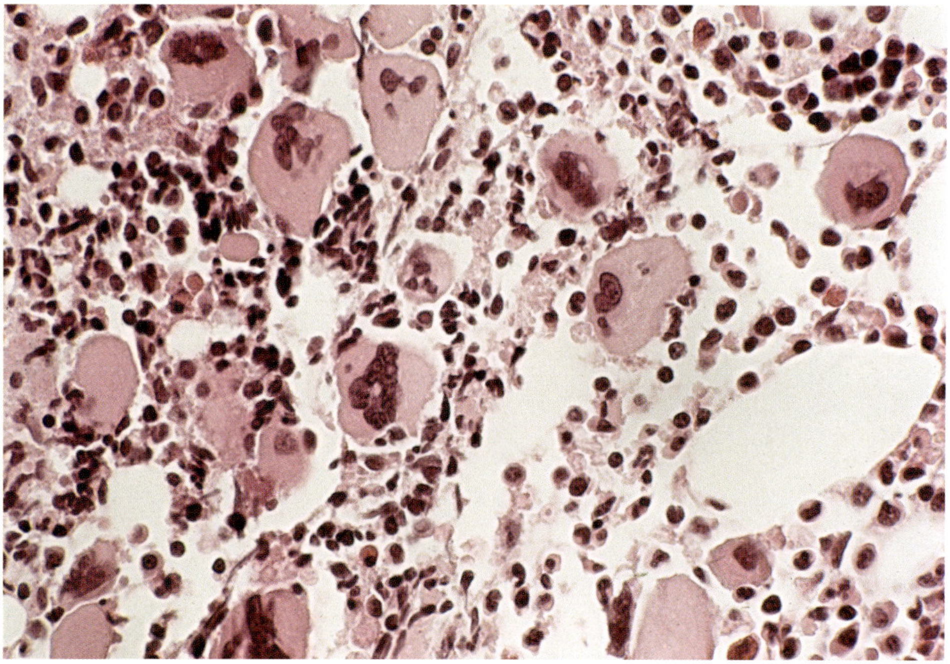

Blood film comments	
Red cell comments	Slight anisocytosis Slight microcytes Slight hypochromasia
White blood cell comments	Neutrophilia
Platelet comments	Thrombocytosis Large and giant platelets

Question 1. What is the differential diagnosis?

Based on the differential diagnosis, the following tests should be requested	
Bone marrow, trephine and cytogenetics	
Bone marrow	A normocellular marrow with an increased number of dysplastic megakaryocytes. Suggestive of essential thrombocythaemia.
Trephine	A mildly hypercellular marrow with increased megakaryopoiesis. There are large, hyperlobulated megakaryocytes present with a tendency to cluster.
Molecular cytogenetics	No abnormality detected. The *JAK2* V617F mutation is detected in 40–50% of cases of essential thrombocythaemia.

Question 2. Are further tests indicated as part of your final report? If so, which tests?

CASE STUDY 42

Case history

A 4-year-old male with pallor, malaise and fever. On examination he is found to have a hepatosplenomegaly and lymphadenopathy.

Analyser data

Parameters	Test Results		Reference Range	
RBC	3.09	× 10^{12}/L	3.96–4.92	× 10^{12}/L
Hb	99	g/L	110–139	g/L
HCT	0.303		0.32–0.39	
MCV	98.1	fL	74–86	fL
MCH	32.0	pg	25.5–30.6	pg
MCHC	327	g/L	310–360	g/L
RDW-SD	43.2	fL	34.6–42.7	fL
RDW-CV	15.2	%	11.9–14.9	%
RETIC CT	4.0	%	0.2–2.0	%
RETIC ABS	123.6	× 10^9/L	20–80	× 10^9/L
WBC	27.4	× 10^9/L	4.7–12.3	× 10^9/L
Plat	206	× 10^9/L	205–457	× 10^9/L

Differential

Parameters	Test Results				Reference Range	
Neutrophil	14.0	%	3.8	× 10^9/L	1.8–7.7	× 10^9/L
Lymphocyte	16.0	%	4.4	× 10^9/L	1.6–5.1	× 10^9/L
Monocyte	42.0	%	11.5	× 10^9/L	0.1–1.0	× 10^9/L
Eosinophil	4.0	%	1.10	× 10^9/L	0.0–0.6	× 10^9/L
Basophil	4	%	1.10	× 10^9/L	0.00–0.10	× 10^9/L
Blast	1	%				
Promyelocyte	1	%				
Myelocyte	13	%				
Band form	5	%				
NRBC	1 / 100 WBC					
ESR	48 mm/h				<5 mm/h	

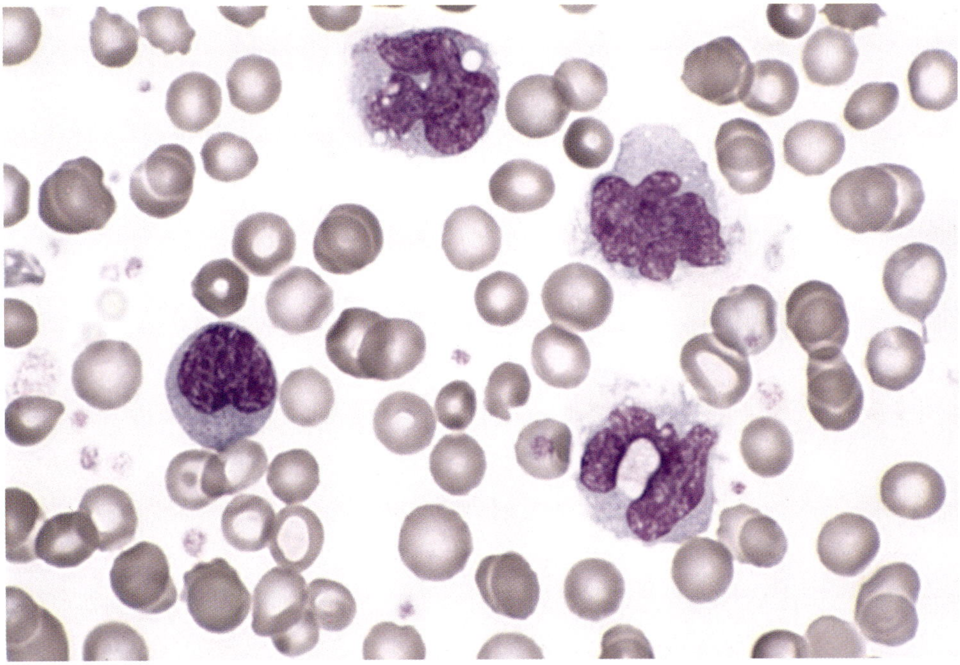

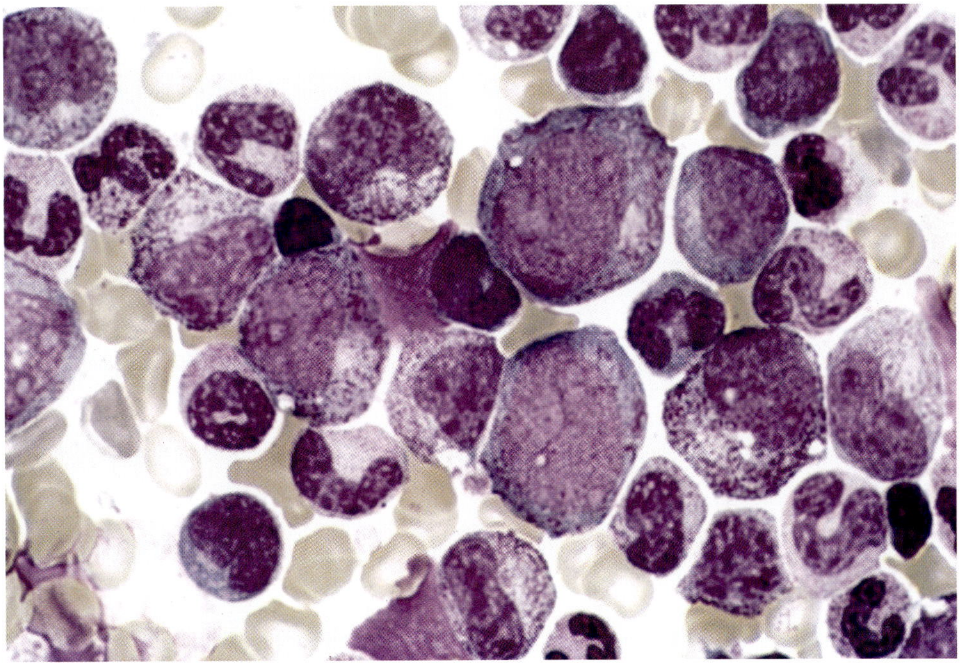

Blood film comments	
Red cell comments	Slight anisocytosis Slight polychromasia Slight rouleaux 1 NRBC / 100 WBC
White blood cell comments	Left shift in the myeloid line Monocytosis Eosinophilia Basophilia 1% blasts Leucoerythroblastic blood film
Platelet comments	Normal in number Large platelets present The MPV and PDW are raised

Question 1. What is the differential diagnosis?

Based on the differential diagnosis, the following tests should be requested	
Bone marrow, cytogenetics, HbF	
Bone marrow	The bone marrow is hypercellular with myeloid hyperplasia and decreased numbers of megakaryocytes.
Cytogenetics	Philadelphia chromosome negative. Monosomy 7 (-7)
HbF	6.4% RR (<1) % (raised for the age of the child).

Question 2. Are further tests indicated as part of your final report? If so, which tests?

CASE STUDY 43

Case history

A 82-year-old female with a history of fever, weight loss and night sweats.

Analyser data				
Parameters	**Test Results**		**Reference Range**	
RBC	3.05	× 10^{12}/L	3.80–5.80	× 10^{12}/L
Hb	90	g/L	115–165	g/L
HCT	0.296		0.37–0.47	
MCV	97.0	fL	80–100	fL
MCH	29.5	pg	26.5–33.0	pg
MCHC	304	g/L	310–360	g/L
RDW-SD	94.0	fL	38.0–48.0	fL
RDW-CV	29.6	%	12.0–14.5	%
RETIC CT				
RETIC ABS				
WBC	169.2	× 10^9/L	3.5–11.0	× 10^9/L
Plat	359	× 10^9/L	150–400	× 10^9/L

Differential						
Parameters	**Test Results**				**Reference Range**	
Neutrophil	28.0	%	47.4	× 10^9/L	1.7–7.0	× 10^9/L
Lymphocyte	5.0	%	8.5	× 10^9/L	1.5–4.0	× 10^9/L
Monocyte	32.0	%	54.1	× 10^9/L	0.1–0.8	× 10^9/L
Eosinophil	1.0	%	1.69	× 10^9/L	0.04–0.44	× 10^9/L
Basophil	0.0	%	0.00	× 10^9/L	0.00–0.20	× 10^9/L
Myelocyte	15	%				
Metamyelocyte	7	%				
Band form	12	%				

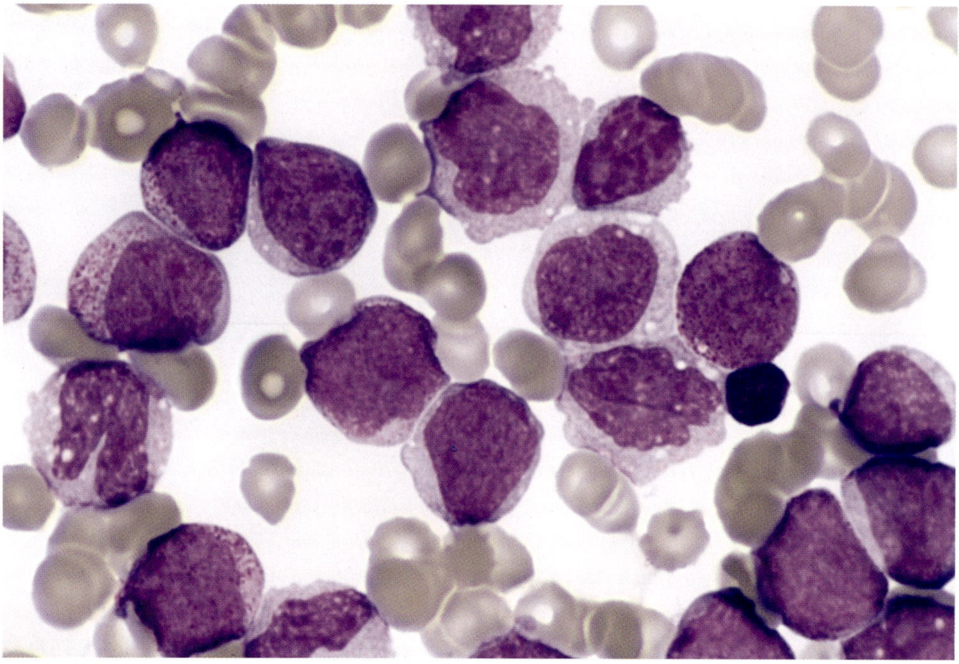

Blood film comments	
Red cell comments	Moderate anisocytosis Slight microcytes Slight macrocytes
White blood cell comments	Neutrophilia Monocytosis Hypogranular and pelgeroid neutrophils
Platelet comments	Large and giant platelets

Question 1. What is the differential diagnosis?

Based on the differential diagnosis, the following tests should be requested	
Bone marrow, trephine, and cytogenetics	
Bone marrow	The bone marrow shows trilineage dysplasia. Dyserythropoiesis, left-shifted dysgranulopoiesis with 3% blasts and dysmegakaryopoiesis. These changes are consistent with the myelodysplastic/myeloproliferative neoplasm chronic myelomonocytic leukaemia Group 1.
Trephine	The trephine shows similar features.
Cytogenetics	−7/del(7q)

Question 2. Are further tests indicated as part of your final report? If so, which tests?

CASE STUDY 44

Case history

An 86-year-old male with recurrent fevers and generally feeling unwell.

Analyser data				
Parameters	**Test Results**		**Reference Range**	
RBC	3.57	× 10^{12}/L	4.50–6.50	× 10^{12}/L
Hb	92	g/L	130–180	g/L
HCT	0.278		0.40–0.54	
MCV	77.9	fL	80–100	fL
MCH	25.8	pg	26.5–33.0	pg
MCHC	331	g/L	310–360	g/L
RDW-SD	63.6	fL	38.0–48.0	fL
RDW-CV	32.7	%	12.0–14.5	%
RETIC CT				
RETIC ABS				
WBC	4.7	× 10^9/L	3.5–11.0	× 10^9/L
Plat	185	× 10^9/L	150–400	× 10^9/L

Differential						
Parameters	**Test Results**				**Reference Range**	
Neutrophil	27.0	%	1.3	× 10^9/L	1.7–7.0	× 10^9/L
Lymphocyte	29.0	%	1.4	× 10^9/L	1.5–4.0	× 10^9/L
Monocyte	31.0	%	1.5	× 10^9/L	0.1–0.8	× 10^9/L
Eosinophil	1.0	%	0.05	× 10^9/L	0.04–0.44	× 10^9/L
Basophil	2.0	%	0.09	× 10^9/L	0.00–0.20	× 10^9/L
Myelocyte	6	%				
Band form	4	%				

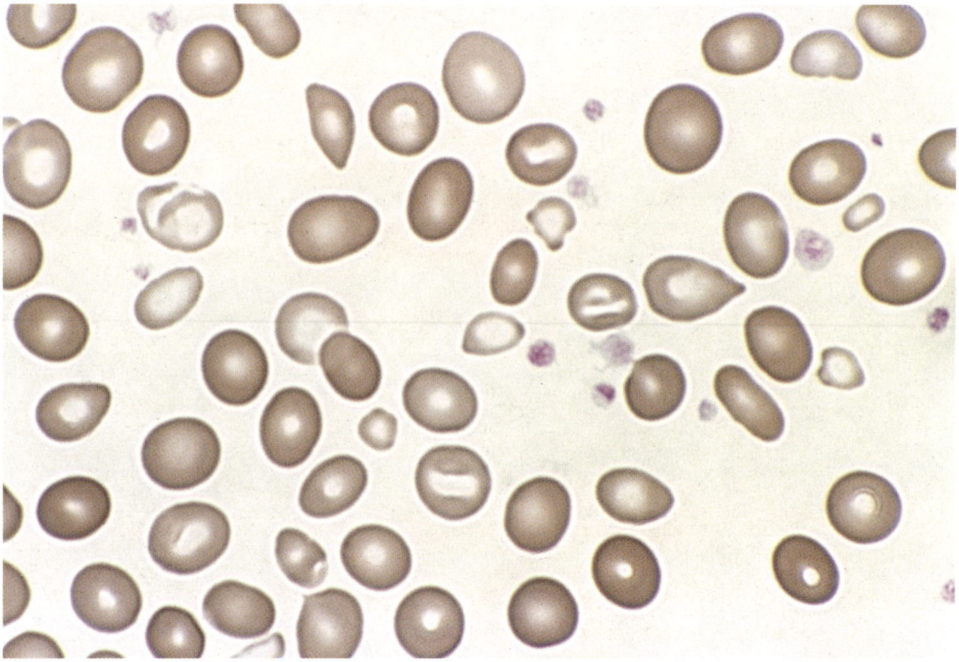

Blood film comments	
Red cell comments	Moderate anisocytosis Slight microcytes Slight hypochromasia Slight macrocytes Dimorphic blood picture
White blood cell comments	Left shift in the myeloid line Monocytosis
Platelet comments	Occasional large platelet

Question 1. What is the differential diagnosis?

Based on the differential diagnosis, the following tests should be requested	
Bone marrow, iron stain and cytogenetics	
Bone marrow	The red cell precursors in the marrow show dysplastic changes such as nuclear budding, multinuclearity, internuclear and intercytoplasmic bridging, as well as megaloblastoid changes. Occasional blast cell (<5%) in the marrow.
Iron stain	Less than 15% of the erythroid precursors are ring sideroblasts.
Cytogenetics	del(20), +8, –5/del(5q), –7/del(7q)

Question 2. Are further tests indicated as part of your final report? If so which tests?

CASE STUDY 45

Case history

A 50-year-old female feeling tired and lethargic.

Analyser data				
Parameters	**Test Results**		**Reference Range**	
RBC	4.41	$\times 10^{12}$/L	3.80–5.80	$\times 10^{12}$/L
Hb	97	g/L	115–165	g/L
HCT	0.334		0.37–0.47	
MCV	75.7	fL	80–100	fL
MCH	22.0	pg	26.5–33.0	pg
MCHC	290	g/L	310–360	g/L
RDW-SD	65.0	fL	38.0–48.0	fL
RDW-CV	24.1	%	12.0–14.5	%
RETIC CT				
RETIC ABS				
WBC	14.3	$\times 10^{9}$/L	3.5–11.0	$\times 10^{9}$/L
Plat	114	$\times 10^{9}$/L	150–400	$\times 10^{9}$/L

Differential						
Parameters	**Test Results**				**Reference Range**	
Neutrophil	84.0	%	12.0	$\times 10^{9}$/L	1.7–7.0	$\times 10^{9}$/L
Lymphocyte	8.0	%	1.2	$\times 10^{9}$/L	1.5–4.0	$\times 10^{9}$/L
Monocyte	6.0	%	0.9	$\times 10^{9}$/L	0.1–0.8	$\times 10^{9}$/L
Eosinophil	1.0	%	0.1	$\times 10^{9}$/L	0.04–0.44	$\times 10^{9}$/L
Basophil	0.0	%	0.00	$\times 10^{9}$/L	0.00–0.20	$\times 10^{9}$/L
Blast	1	%				
NRBC	6 / 100 WBC					

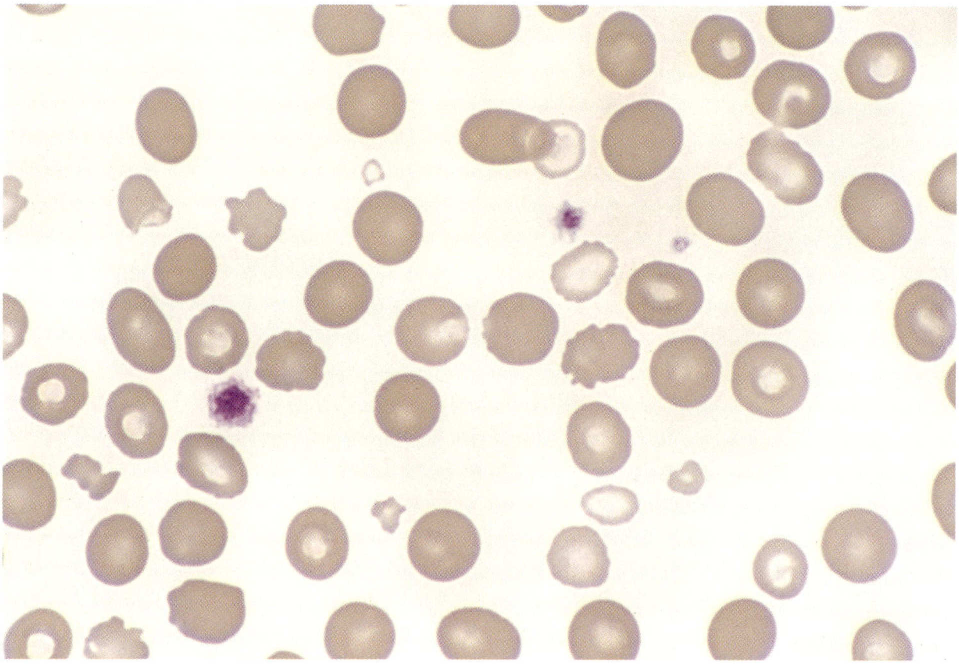

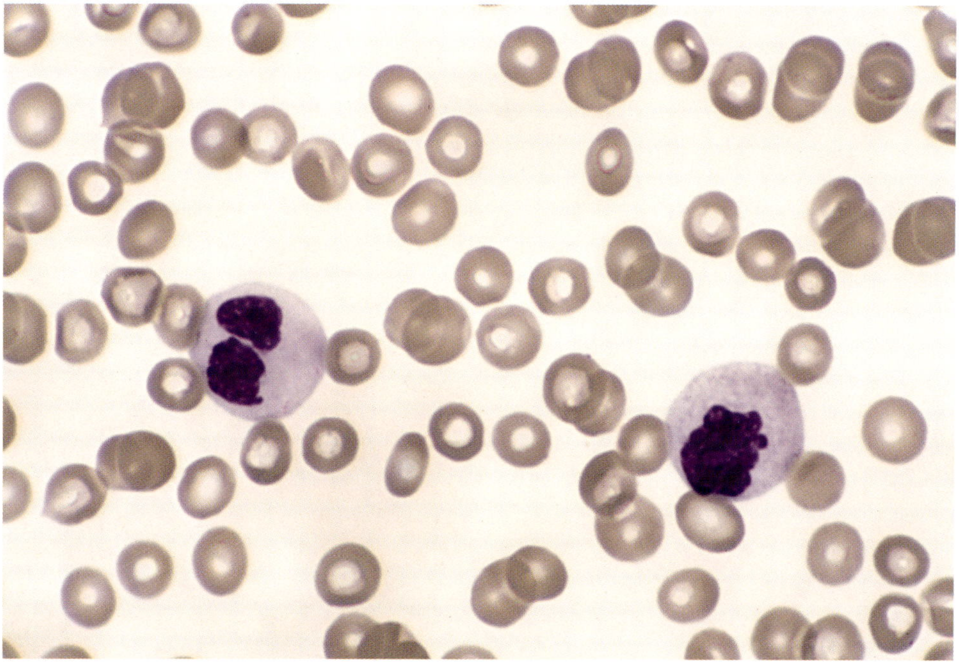

Blood film comments	
Red cell comments	Marked anisocytosis Moderate microcytes Moderate hypochromasia Moderate macrocytes Slight polychromasia Dimorphic blood film 6 NRBC / 100 WBC Many of the NRBCs show dysplastic nuclei
White blood cell comments	Neutrophilia Marked hypogranular and agranular neutrophils Marked pelgeroid neutrophils 1% Blasts
Platelet comments	Large and giant platelets

Question 1. What is the differential diagnosis?

Based on the differential diagnosis, the following tests should be requested	
Bone marrow, iron stain and cytogenetics	
Bone marrow	Both the peripheral blood film and bone marrow show marked dysplastic changes in all three cell lines. The red cell precursors in the marrow show dysplastic changes such as nuclear budding, multinuclearity, internuclear and intercytoplasmic bridging, as well as megaloblastoid changes. The neutrophils are hypogranular and agranular with pelgeroid features. There is an occasional blast cell (<5%). The megakaryocytes show dysplastic features such as micromegakaryocytes with small hypolobulated nuclei as well as hypersegmented megakaryocytes.
Iron stain	Approximately 15% of the erythroid precursors are ring sideroblasts.
Cytogenetics	del(20), +8, −5/del(5q), −7/del(7q)

Question 2. Are further tests indicated as part of your final report? If so, which tests?

CASE STUDY 46

Case history

A 7-year-old child with severe tonsillitis.

Analyser data

Parameters	Test Results		Reference Range	
RBC	4.17	× 10^{12}/L	3.96–4.92	× 10^{12}/L
Hb	114	g/L	110–139	g/L
HCT	0.351		0.32–0.39	
MCV	84.2	fL	74–86	fL
MCH	27.3	pg	25.5–30.6	pg
MCHC	325	g/L	310–360	g/L
RDW-SD	36.7	fL	34.6–42.7	fL
RDW-CV	12.6	%	11.9–14.9	%
RETIC CT				
RETIC ABS				
WBC	10.3	× 10^9/L	4.7–12.3	× 10^9/L
Plat	150	× 10^9/L	205–457	× 10^9/L

Differential

Parameters	Test Results				Reference Range	
Neutrophil	20.0	%	2.1	× 10^9/L	1.8–7.7	× 10^9/L
Lymphocyte	39.0	%	4.0	× 10^9/L	1.6–5.1	× 10^9/L
Monocyte	4.0	%	0.4	× 10^9/L	0.1–1.0	× 10^9/L
Eosinophil	0.0	%	0.00	× 10^9/L	0.00–0.06	× 10^9/L
Basophil	0.0	%	0.00		0.00–0.10	× 10^9/L
Reactive lymphocyte	37	%				

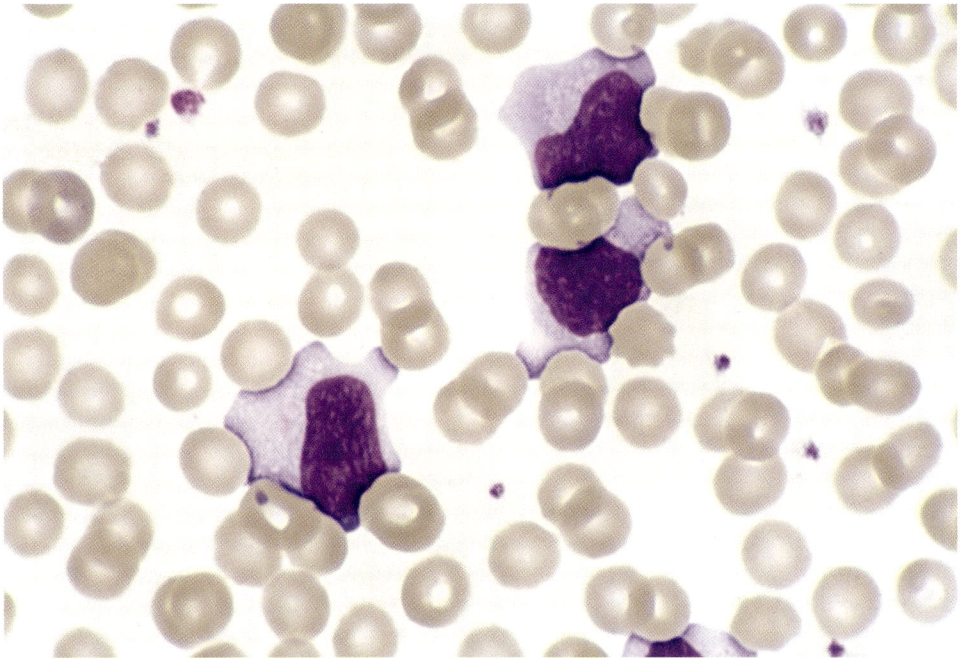

Blood film comments	
Red cell comments	Normal in number and morphology
White blood cell comments	37% reactive lymphocytes
Platelet comments	Thrombocytopenia

Question 1. What is the differential diagnosis?

Based on the differential diagnosis, the following tests should be requested		
Monospot test (screening test for infectious mononucleosis) and Epstein Barr virus (EBV) antibody		
Monospot test	Positive	
Epstein Barr virus	Epstein Barr NA IgG antibody Epstein Barr VCA IgG antibody Epstein Barr VCA IgM antibody Epstein Barr VCA IgG avidity index	Negative Positive Positive 79
EBV VCA IgM antibody appears in both primary infection and reactivation of EBV. EBV VCA IgG antibody appears early in primary infection and in most cases should last for life. Low avidity IgG antibody only appears in primary EBV infection and increases to approximately 80% by 6 months. EB NA IgG appears after about 6 months and in most cases should last for life. The combination of low EBV VCA IgG avidity with positive EBV VCA IgM and negative EB NA IgG is 100% specific for the diagnosis of primary EBV infection.		

Question 2. Are further tests indicated as part of your final report? If so, which tests?

CASE STUDY 47

Case history
A 31-year-old male presents with a superficial eruption of macular transparent vesicles on his back.

Analyser data				
Parameters	**Test Results**		**Reference Range**	
RBC	5.33	$\times 10^{12}$/L	4.50–6.50	$\times 10^{12}$/L
Hb	164	g/L	130–180	g/L
HCT	0.473		0.40–0.54	
MCV	88.7	fL	80–100	fL
MCH	30.8	pg	26.5–33.0	pg
MCHC	347	g/L	310–360	g/L
RDW-SD	39.7	fL	38.0–48.0	fL
RDW-CV	14.1	%	12.0–14.5	%
RETIC CT				
RETIC ABS				
WBC	10.5	$\times 10^9$/L	3.5–11.0	$\times 10^9$/L
Plat	148	$\times 10^9$/L	150–400	$\times 10^9$/L

Differential						
Parameters	**Test Results**				**Reference Range**	
Neutrophil	41.0	%	4.3	$\times 10^9$/L	1.7–7.0	$\times 10^9$/L
Lymphocyte	24.0	%	2.5	$\times 10^9$/L	1.5–4.0	$\times 10^9$/L
Monocyte	0.0	%	0.0	$\times 10^9$/L	0.1–0.8	$\times 10^9$/L
Eosinophil	0.0	%	0.0	$\times 10^9$/L	0.04–0.44	$\times 10^9$/L
Basophil	0.0	%	0.0	$\times 10^9$/L	0.00–0.20	$\times 10^9$/L
Band form	15	%				
Reactive lymphocyte	20	%				

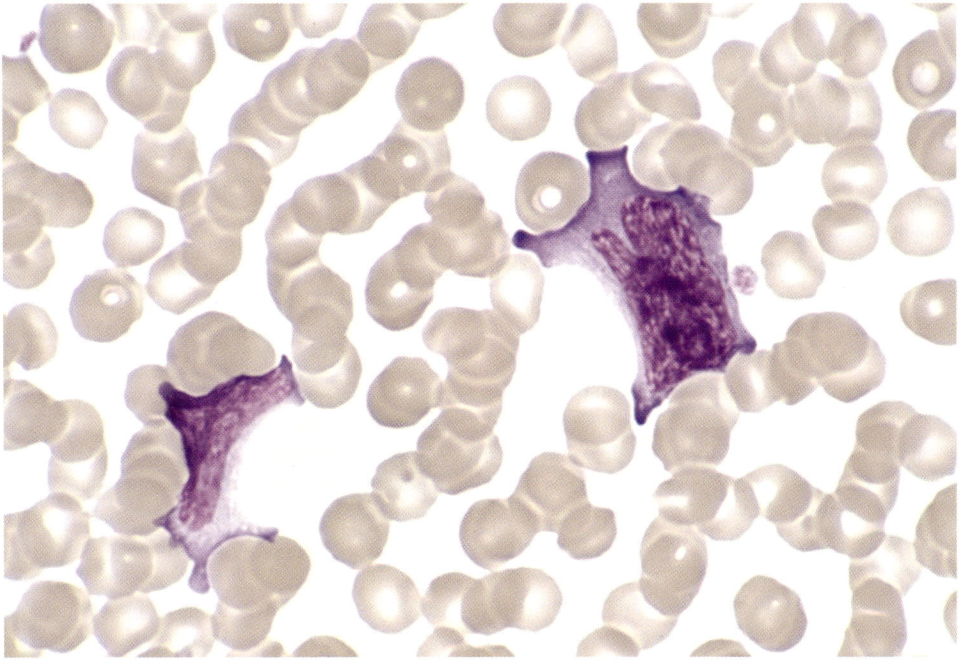

Blood film comments	
Red cell comments	Normal in number and morphology
White blood cell comments	Left shift in the myeloid line 20% reactive lymphocytes
Platelet comments	Thrombocytopenia

Question 1. What is the differential diagnosis?

Based on the differential diagnosis, the following tests should be requested		
Monospot test (screening test for infectious mononucleosis) and viral studies		
Monospot test	Negative.	
Viral studies	Varicella zoster IgG antibody Varicella zoster IgM antibody	Positive Positive
Consistent with recent infection of varicella zoster or chicken pox.		

Question 2. Are further tests indicated as part of your final report? If so, which tests?

CASE STUDY 48

Case history

A 63-year-old male, returning from Southeast Asia, presents with an acute febrile illness.

Analyser data				
Parameters	**Test Results**		**Reference Range**	
RBC	3.57	× 10^{12}/L	4.50–6.50	× 10^{12}/L
Hb	110	g/L	130–180	g/L
HCT	0.331		0.40–0.54	
MCV	92.7	fL	80–100	fL
MCH	30.8	pg	26.5–33.0	pg
MCHC	332	g/L	310–360	g/L
RDW-SD	66.1	fL	38.0–48.0	fL
RDW-CV	19.5	%	12.0–14.5	%
RETIC CT				
RETIC ABS				
WBC	0.43	× 10^9/L	3.5–11.0	× 10^9/L
Plat	14	× 10^9/L	150–400	× 10^9/L

Differential						
Parameters	**Test Results**				**Reference Range**	
Neutrophil	36.0	%	0.2	× 10^9/L	1.7–7.0	× 10^9/L
Lymphocyte	35.0	%	0.2	× 10^9/L	1.5–4.0	× 10^9/L
Monocyte	6.0	%	0.03	× 10^9/L	0.1–0.8	× 10^9/L
Eosinophil	0.0	%	0.00	× 10^9/L	0.04–0.44	× 10^9/L
Basophil	1.0	%	0.00	× 10^9/L	0.00–0.20	× 10^9/L
Myelocyte	14	%				
Türk cell	8	%				
NRBC	16 / 100 WBC					
ESR	87 mm/h				<20 mm/h	

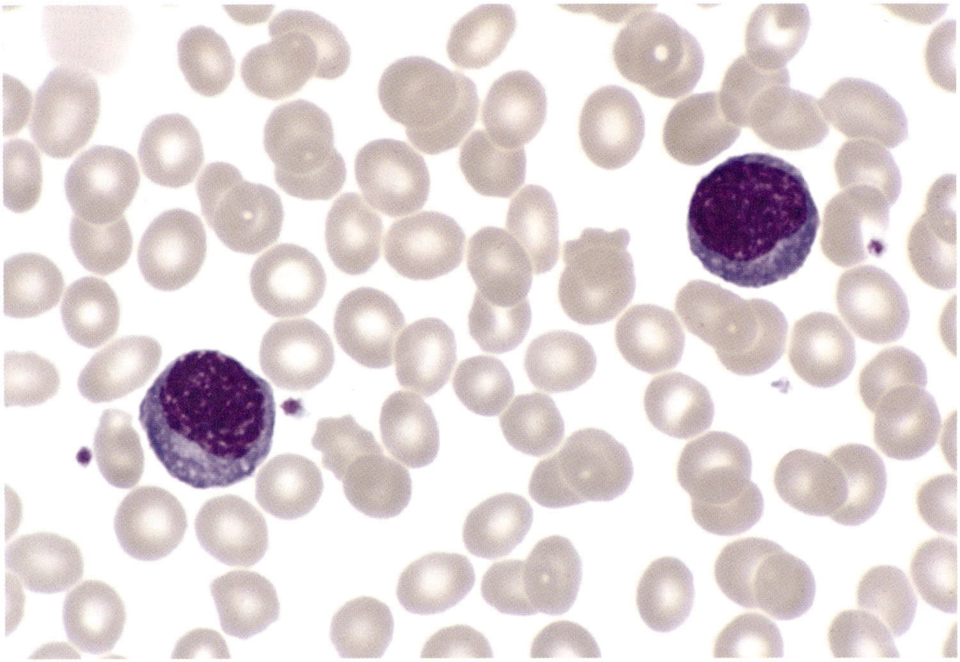

Blood film comments	
Red cell comments	Reduced in number Moderate rouleaux 16 NRBC / 100 WBC
White blood cell comments	Left shift in the myeloid line Leucopenia 8% Türk cells
Platelet comments	Marked thrombocytopenia

Question 1. What is the differential diagnosis?

Based on the differential diagnosis, the following tests should be requested		
Thick and thin films for malaria Monospot screening test for infectious mononucleosis Viral studies including screening for dengue fever		
Thick and thin films for malaria	Negative	
Monospot test	Negative	
Viral studies	Dengue fever IgG antibody Dengue fever IgM antibody	Negative. Positive (suggestive of primary dengue infection)
The presence of Türk cells on the blood film is highly suggestive of dengue fever.		

Question 2. Are further tests indicated as part of your final report? If so, which tests?

CASE STUDY 49

Case history

A 6-week-old infant with a cough admitted to the intensive care ward.

Analyser data				
Parameters	**Test Results**		**Reference Range**	
RBC	3.37	$\times 10^{12}$/L	3.38–3.94	$\times 10^{12}$/L
Hb	102	g/L	102–130	g/L
HCT	0.296		0.30–0.38	
MCV	87.8	fL	84–98	fL
MCH	30.3	pg	29.0–33.8	pg
MCHC	345	g/L	310–360	g/L
RDW-SD	42.4	fL	39.9–56.6	fL
RDW-CV	13.7	%	12.6–16.0	%
RETIC CT				
RETIC ABS				
WBC	16.2	$\times 10^9$/L	6.4–12.1	$\times 10^9$/L
Plat	643	$\times 10^9$/L	270–645	$\times 10^9$/L

Differential						
Parameters	**Test Results**				**Reference Range**	
Neutrophil	13.1	%	2.1	$\times 10^9$/L	0.8–4.9	$\times 10^9$/L
Lymphocyte	76.7	%	12.4	$\times 10^9$/L	3.8–7.6	$\times 10^9$/L
Monocyte	5.1	%	0.8	$\times 10^9$/L	0.3–1.2	$\times 10^9$/L
Eosinophil	4.6	%	0.75	$\times 10^9$/L	0.1–0.8	$\times 10^9$/L
Basophil	0.5	%	0.08	$\times 10^9$/L	0.00–0.20	$\times 10^9$/L

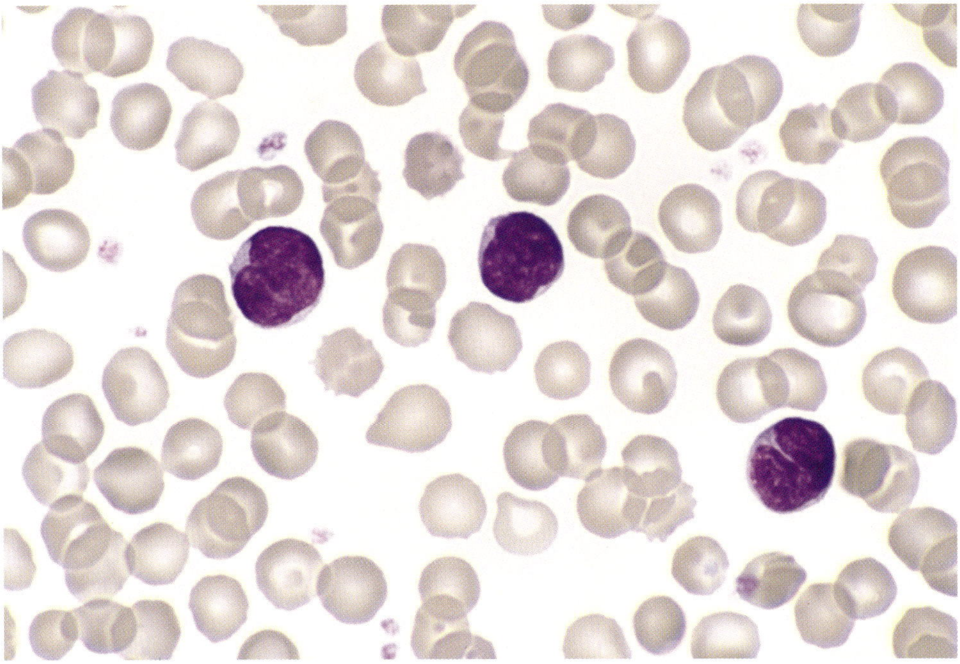

Blood film comments	
Red cell comments	Normal in number and morphology
White blood cell comments	Lymphocytosis Many of the lymphocytes have cleaved nuclei
Platelet comments	Normal in number and morphology

Question 1. What is the differential diagnosis?

Based on the differential diagnosis, the following tests should be requested
Pertussis PCR
Pertussis PCR Nasopharyngeal swabs were positive for *Bordetella pertussis*. Given the clinical notes no further testing was performed.
Morphologically, the lymphocytes of *Bordetella pertussis* classically have cleaved nuclei. Their presence on the blood film should be observed and reported to the treating clinician urgently so that the relevant antibiotics can be commenced if clinically indicated. *Pertussis* PCR is usually performed weekly so it can take some time for a result to become available.

Question 2. Are further tests indicated as part of your final report? If so, which tests?

CASE STUDY 50

Case history

An 81-year-old female having a routine full blood count.

Analyser data				
Parameters	**Test Results**		**Reference Range**	
RBC	4.54	$\times 10^{12}$/L	3.80–5.80	$\times 10^{12}$/L
Hb	108	g/L	115–165	g/L
HCT	0.379		0.37–0.47	
MCV	83.5	fL	80–100	fL
MCH	23.8	pg	26.5–33.0	pg
MCHC	285	g/L	310–360	g/L
RDW-SD	48.7	fL	38.0–48.0	fL
RDW-CV	14.7	%	12.0–14.5	%
RETIC CT				
RETIC ABS				
WBC	88.2	$\times 10^{9}$/L	3.5–11.0	$\times 10^{9}$/L
Plat	393	$\times 10^{9}$/L	150–400	$\times 10^{9}$/L

Differential						
Parameters	**Test Results**				**Reference Range**	
Neutrophil	9.9	%	8.8	$\times 10^{9}$/L	1.7–7.0	$\times 10^{9}$/L
Lymphocyte	88.1	%	77.6	$\times 10^{9}$/L	1.5–4.0	$\times 10^{9}$/L
Monocyte	1.5	%	1.3	$\times 10^{9}$/L	0.1–0.8	$\times 10^{9}$/L
Eosinophil	0.2	%	0.2	$\times 10^{9}$/L	0.04–0.44	$\times 10^{9}$/L
Basophil	0.3	%	0.3	$\times 10^{9}$/L	0.00–0.20	$\times 10^{9}$/L

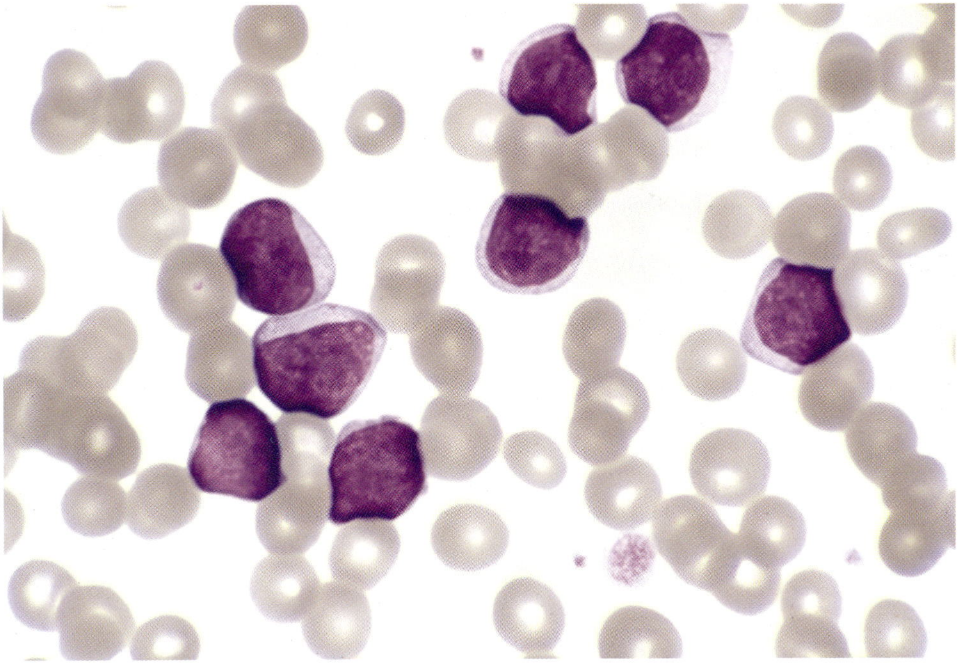

Blood film comments	
Red cell comments	Slight anisocytosis Slight microcytes Slight hypochromasia Iron studies may be indicated
White blood cell comments	Lymphocytosis Smudge cells
Platelet comments	Normal in number and morphology

Question 1. What is the differential diagnosis?

Based on the differential diagnosis, the following tests should be requested	
Bone marrow, trephine, immunophenotyping and cytogenetics	
Bone marrow	Hypercellular marrow with an infiltrate of small lymphocytes with clumped chromatin and scanty cytoplasm. Less than 2% prolymphocytes. Occasional smudge cell. Bone marrow trephine as above.
Immunophenotype	SIg^+ (weak), $CD5^+$, $CD10^-$, $CD19^+$, $CD20^+$, $CD22^+$, $CD23^+$, $CD43^+$, $CD79a^+$
Cytogenetics	Common abnormalities include del(13q), +12, del(11q) and del(17p)

Question 2. Are further tests indicated as part of your final report? If so, which tests?

CASE STUDY 51

Case history

A 76-year-old male presents with a splenomegaly.

Analyser data				
Parameters	**Test Results**		**Reference Range**	
RBC	4.00	$\times 10^{12}/L$	4.50–6.50	$\times 10^{12}/L$
Hb	125	g/L	130–180	g/L
HCT	0.375		0.40–0.54	
MCV	91.3	fL	80–100	fL
MCH	27.0	pg	26.5–33.0	pg
MCHC	335	g/L	310–360	g/L
RDW-SD	48.7	fL	38.0–48.0	fL
RDW-CV	15.2	%	12.0–14.5	%
RETIC CT				
RETIC ABS				
WBC	503.3	$\times 10^9/L$	3.5–11.0	$\times 10^9/L$
Plat	146	$\times 10^9/L$	150–400	$\times 10^9/L$

Differential						
Parameters	**Test Results**				**Reference Range**	
Neutrophil	2.0	%	10.1	$\times 10^9/L$	1.7–7.0	$\times 10^9/L$
Lymphocyte	10.0	%	50.3	$\times 10^9/L$	1.5–4.0	$\times 10^9/L$
Monocyte	3.0	%	15.1	$\times 10^9/L$	0.1–0.8	$\times 10^9/L$
Eosinophil	0.0	%	0.0	$\times 10^9/L$	0.04–0.44	$\times 10^9/L$
Basophil	0.0	%	0.0	$\times 10^9/L$	0.00–0.20	$\times 10^9/L$
Prolymphocyte	85	%				

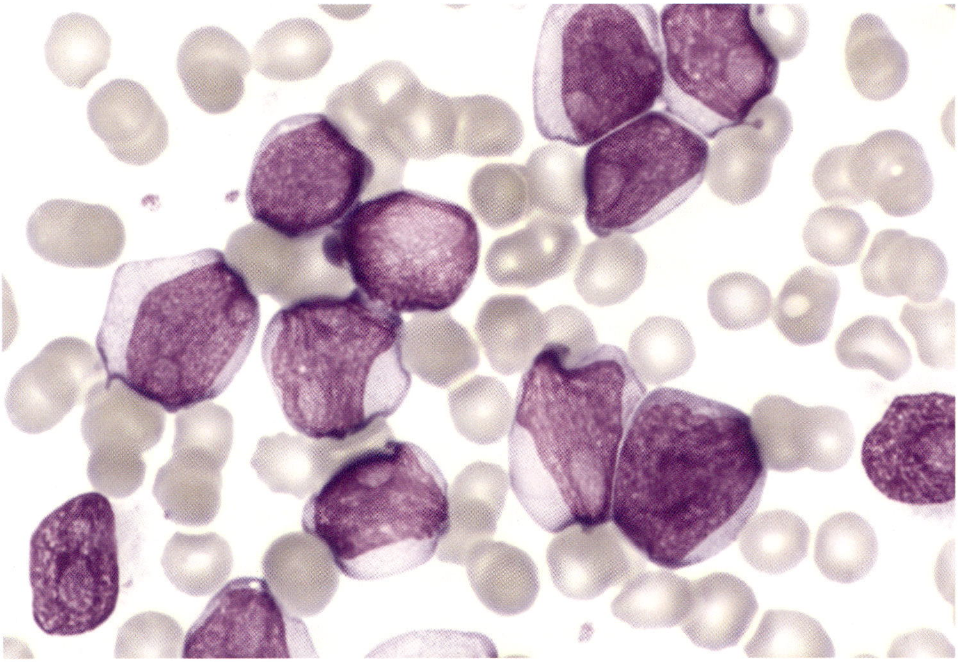

Blood film comments	
Red cell comments	Slight anisocytosis
White blood cell comments	85% prolymphocytes
Platelet comments	Thrombocytopenia

Question 1. What is the differential diagnosis?

Based on the differential diagnosis, the following tests should be requested	
Bone marrow, trephine, immunophenotyping and cytogenetics	
Bone marrow	The marrow shows an infiltrate of prolymphocytes with round nuclei, condensed chromatin pattern and a single large nucleolus. Bone marrow trephine as above.
Immunophenotype	SIg^+, $CD5^{-/+}$, $CD19^+$, $CD20^+$, $CD22^+$, $CD23^{-/+}$, $CD79a^+$
Cytogenetics	Karyotypes are often complex with abnormalities such as del(17p), del(13)(q14), del(11q), and less commonly +12.

Question 2. Are further tests indicated as part of your final report? If so, which tests?

CASE STUDY 52

Case history

A male 84 years of age presents with lassitude; on examination he is found to have an enlarged spleen.

Analyser data

Parameters	Test Results		Reference Range	
RBC	4.48	$\times 10^{12}/L$	4.50–6.50	$\times 10^{12}/L$
Hb	114	g/L	130–180	g/L
HCT	0.374		0.40–0.54	
MCV	83.5	fL	80–100	fL
MCH	25.4	pg	26.5–33.0	pg
MCHC	305	g/L	310–360	g/L
RDW-SD	48.2	fL	38.0–48.0	fL
RDW-CV	14.6	%	12.0–14.5	%
RETIC CT				
RETIC ABS				
WBC	13.5	$\times 10^9/L$	3.5–11.0	$\times 10^9/L$
Plat	258	$\times 10^9/L$	150–400	$\times 10^9/L$

Differential

Parameters	Test Results				Reference Range	
Neutrophil	58.0	%	7.8	$\times 10^9/L$	1.7–7.0	$\times 10^9/L$
Lymphocyte	15.0	%	2.0	$\times 10^9/L$	1.5–4.0	$\times 10^9/L$
Monocyte	4.0	%	0.5	$\times 10^9/L$	0.1–0.8	$\times 10^9/L$
Eosinophil	0.0	%	0.00	$\times 10^9/L$	0.04–0.44	$\times 10^9/L$
Basophil	0.0	%	0.00	$\times 10^9/L$	0.00–0.20	$\times 10^9/L$
Lymphoma cell	23	%				

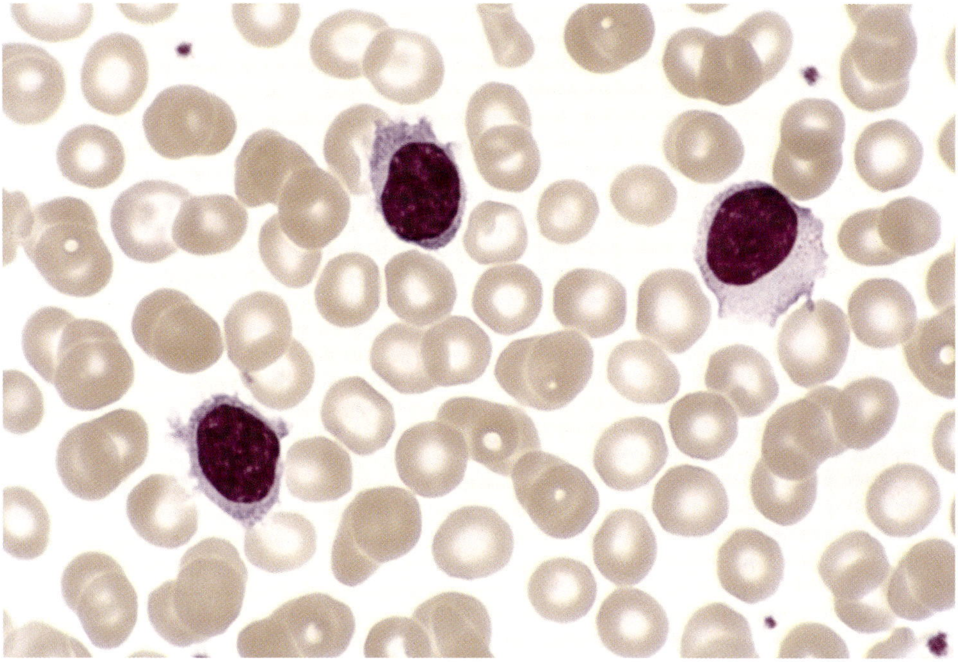

Blood film comments	
Red cell comments	Slight anisocytosis Slight microcytes Slight hypochromasia Iron studies may be indicated
White blood cell comments	23% lymphoma cells
Platelet comments	Normal in number and morphology

Question 1. What is the differential diagnosis?

Based on the differential diagnosis, the following tests should be requested	
Bone marrow, trephine, immunophenotyping and cytogenetics	
Bone marrow	The marrow is infiltrated with mature lymphocytes with oval nuclei, basophilic cytoplasm with thin, short villi concentrated towards one pole of the cell. Bone marrow trephine as above.
Immunophenotype	SIg^{+}, $CD5^{-}$, $CD10^{-}$, $CD19^{+}$, $CD20^{+}$, $CD22^{+}$, $CD23^{-}$, $CD43^{-}$, $CD79a^{+}$
Cytogenetics	Deletions and rearrangements of 7q, +3q, and t(11;14)(q13;q32)

Question 2. Are further tests indicated as part of your final report? If so, which tests?

CASE STUDY 53

Case history

A 58-year-old female with symptoms of weakness and fatigue.

Analyser data				
Parameters	**Test Results**		**Reference Range**	
RBC	4.13	$\times 10^{12}/L$	3.80–5.80	$\times 10^{12}/L$
Hb	127	g/L	115–165	g/L
HCT	0.388		0.37–0.47	
MCV	93.9	fL	80–100	fL
MCH	30.8	pg	26.5–33.0	pg
MCHC	327	g/L	310–360	g/L
RDW-SD	44.7	fL	38.0–48.0	fL
RDW-CV	12.6	%	12.0–14.5	%
RETIC CT				
RETIC ABS				
WBC	85.2	$\times 10^9/L$	3.5–11.0	$\times 10^9/L$
Plat	127	$\times 10^9/L$	150–400	$\times 10^9/L$

Differential						
Parameters	**Test Results**				**Reference Range**	
Neutrophil	5.0	%	4.3	$\times 10^9/L$	1.7–7.0	$\times 10^9/L$
Lymphocyte	10.0	%	8.52	$\times 10^9/L$	1.5–4.0	$\times 10^9/L$
Monocyte	0.0	%	0.00	$\times 10^9/L$	0.1–0.8	$\times 10^9/L$
Eosinophil	0.0	%	0.00	$\times 10^9/L$	0.04–0.44	$\times 10^9/L$
Basophil	0.0	%	0.00	$\times 10^9/L$	0.00–0.20	$\times 10^9/L$
Hairy cell	85	%				

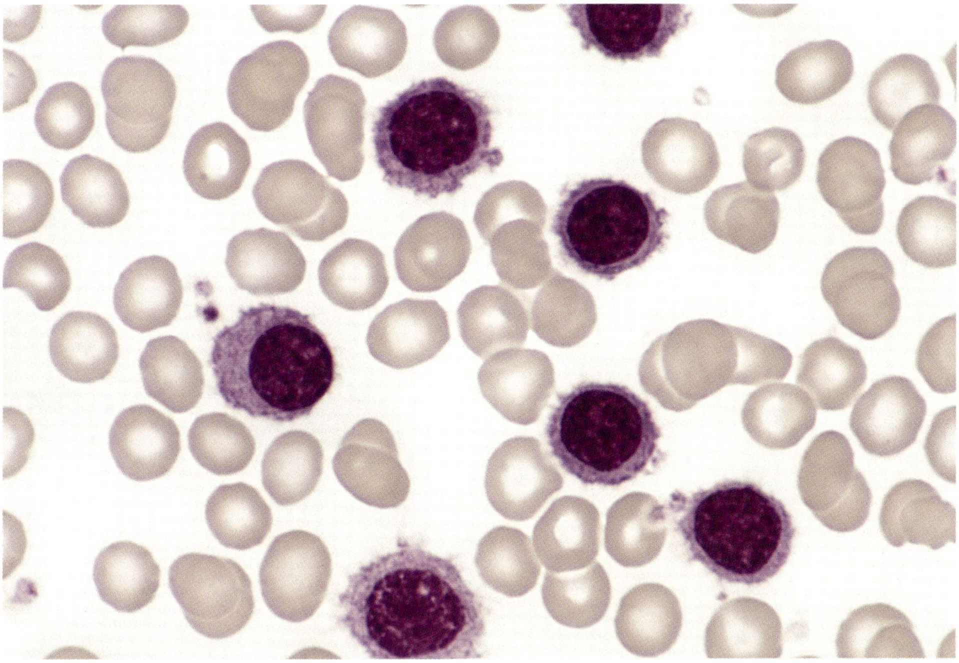

Blood film comments	
Red cell comments	Normal in number and morphology
White blood cell comments	85% hairy cells
Platelet comments	Thrombocytopenia

Question 1. What is the differential diagnosis?

Based on the differential diagnosis, the following tests should be requested	
Bone marrow, trephine, immunophenotyping and cytogenetics	
Bone marrow	The marrow is infiltrated with lymphocytes that have a centrally placed nucleus with many hair-like projections around the entire circumference of the cell. The trephine shows an infiltrate of lymphocyte nuclei surrounded by halos of pale-staining cytoplasm.
Immunophenotype	$CD19^+$, $CD20^+$, $CD22^+$, $CD103^{+/-}$, $CD11c^+$, $CD25^-$ Consistent with the variant form of hairy cell leukaemia.
Cytogenetics	No specific abnormalities. Complex abnormalities involving 14q32 (*IGH*) or 8q24 (*MYC*) and deletions of 17p (*TP53*)

Question 2. Are further tests indicated as part of your final report? If so, which tests?

CASE STUDY 54

Case history

A 52-year-old male presents with lymphadenopathy and splenomegaly.

Analyser data				
Parameters	**Test Results**		**Reference Range**	
RBC	2.54	$\times 10^{12}$/L	4.50–6.50	$\times 10^{12}$/L
Hb	72	g/L	130–180	g/L
HCT	0.238		0.40–0.54	
MCV	93.7	fL	80–100	fL
MCH	28.3	pg	26.5–33.0	pg
MCHC	303	g/L	310–360	g/L
RDW-SD	47.6	fL	38.0–48.0	fL
RDW-CV	14.3	%	12.0–14.5	%
RETIC CT				
RETIC ABS				
WBC	61.1	$\times 10^9$/L	3.5–11.0	$\times 10^9$/L
Plat	10	$\times 10^9$/L	150–400	$\times 10^9$/L

Differential						
Parameters	**Test Results**				**Reference Range**	
Neutrophil	1.0	%	0.6	$\times 10^9$/L	1.7–7.0	$\times 10^9$/L
Lymphocyte	15.0	%	9.2	$\times 10^9$/L	1.5–4.0	$\times 10^9$/L
Monocyte	0.0	%	0.0	$\times 10^9$/L	0.1–0.8	$\times 10^9$/L
Eosinophil	2.0	%	1.22	$\times 10^9$/L	0.04–0.44	$\times 10^9$/L
Basophil	0.0	%	0.0	$\times 10^9$/L	0.00–0.20	$\times 10^9$/L
Lymphoma cell	82	%				
ESR	53 mm/h				<20 mm/h	

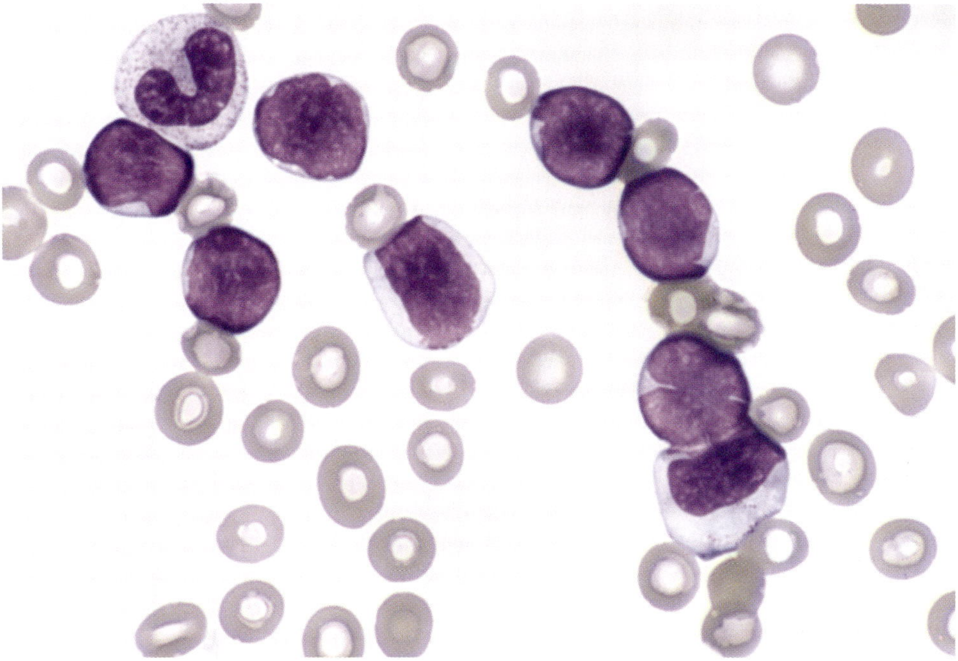

Blood film comments	
Red cell comments	Slight rouleaux
White blood cell comments	82% lymphoma cells
Platelet comments	Thrombocytopenia

Question 1. What is the differential diagnosis?

Based on the differential diagnosis, the following tests should be requested	
Bone marrow, trephine, immunophenotyping and cytogenetics	
Bone marrow	The marrow is infiltrated with large lymphoid cells with round to oval nuclei, one to three nucleoli and a narrow border of pale blue cytoplasm. An initial impression of these cells is that they resemble blasts. Until immunophenotyping has been performed confirming that they are in fact lymphoma cells, one could describe them as 'atypical' lymphoid cells. Post immunophenotyping they should be counted as lymphoma cells. Bone marrow trephine as above.
Immunophenotype	SIg^+, $CD5^-$, $CD10^+$, $CD19^+$, $CD20^+$, $CD79a^+$, $CD22^+$, $CD43^-$, $CD23^+$, $BCL2^+$, $BCL6^+$
Cytogenetics	t(14;18)(q32;q21), t(3;14)(q27;q32), t(3;22)(q27;q11), t(2;3)(p12;q27)

Question 2. Are further tests indicated as part of your final report? If so, which tests?

CASE STUDY 55

Case history

A 79-year-old male with lymphadenopathy and hepatosplenomegaly for investigation.

Analyser data

Parameters	Test Results		Reference Range	
RBC	4.28	× 10^{12}/L	4.50–6.50	× 10^{12}/L
Hb	121	g/L	130–180	g/L
HCT	0.366		0.40–0.54	
MCV	85.5	fL	80–100	fL
MCH	28.3	pg	26.5–33.0	pg
MCHC	331	g/L	310–360	g/L
RDW-SD	47.0	fL	38.0–48.0	fL
RDW-CV	14.3	%	12.0–14.5	%
RETIC CT				
RETIC ABS				
WBC	32.2	× 10^9/L	3.5–11.0	× 10^9/L
Plat	48	× 10^9/L	150–400	× 10^9/L

Differential

Parameters	Test Results				Reference Range	
Neutrophil	65.0	%	20.9	× 10^9/L	1.7–7.0	× 10^9/L
Lymphocyte	9.0	%	2.9	× 10^9/L	1.5–4.0	× 10^9/L
Monocyte	14.0	%	4.50	× 10^9/L	0.1–0.8	× 10^9/L
Eosinophil	0.0	%	0.00	× 10^9/L	0.04–0.44	× 10^9/L
Basophil	0.0	%	0.00	× 10^9/L	0.00–0.20	× 10^9/L
Lymphoma cell	12.0	%				
NRBC	2 / 100 WBC					
ESR	61 mm/h				<20 mm/h	

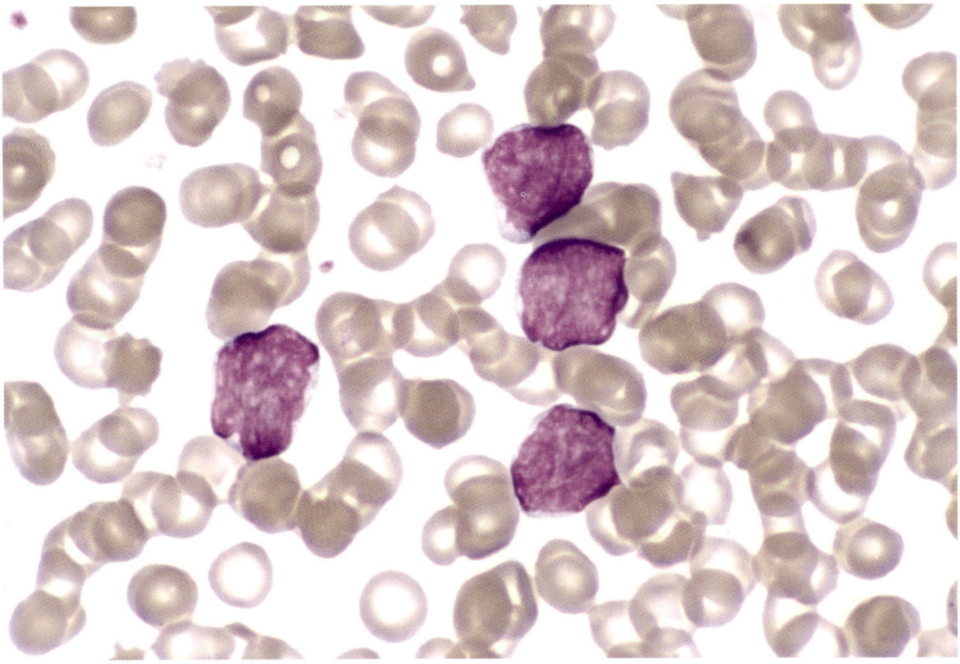

Blood film comments	
Red cell comments	Slight rouleaux 2 NRBC / 100 WBC
White blood cell comments	12% lymphoma cells
Platelet comments	Thrombocytopenia

Question 1. What is the differential diagnosis?

Based on the differential diagnosis, the following tests should be requested	
Bone marrow, trephine, immunophenotyping and cytogenetics	
Bone marrow	Patchy infiltrate of small to medium sized lymphoid cells with irregular shaped nuclei, dispersed chromatin pattern and inconspicuous nucleoli. Bone marrow trephine as above.
Immunophenotype	SIg^{+}, $CD5^{+}$, $CD10^{-}$, $CD19^{+}$, $CD20^{+}$, $CD22^{+}$, $CD23^{-/+}$, $CD43^{+}$, cyclin $D1^{+}$, $BLC2^{+}$, $BLC6^{-}$
Cytogenetics	t(11;14)(q13;q32)

Question 2. Are further tests indicated as part of your final report? If so, which tests?

CASE STUDY 56

Case history

A 13-year-old male presents with a large mass on the left-hand side of his face.

Analyser data				
Parameters	**Test Results**		**Reference Range**	
RBC	5.27	× 10^{12}/L	4.50–6.50	× 10^{12}/L
Hb	157	g/L	130–180	g/L
HCT	0.418		0.40–0.54	
MCV	79.3	fL	80–100	fL
MCH	29.8	pg	26.5–33.0	pg
MCHC	359	g/L	310–360	g/L
RDW-SD	47.6	fL	38.0–48.0	fL
RDW-CV	14.3	%	12.0–14.5	%
RETIC CT				
RETIC ABS				
WBC	6.4	× 10^9/L	3.5–11.0	× 10^9/L
Plat	37	× 10^9/L	150–400	× 10^9/L

Differential						
Parameters	**Test Results**				**Reference Range**	
Neutrophil	23.0	%	1.5	× 10^9/L	1.7–7.0	× 10^9/L
Lymphocyte	45.0	%	2.9	× 10^9/L	1.5–4.0	× 10^9/L
Monocyte	20.0	%	1.27	× 10^9/L	0.1–0.8	× 10^9/L
Eosinophil	1.0	%	0.06	× 10^9/L	0.04–0.44	× 10^9/L
Basophil	0.0	%	0.00	× 10^9/L	0.00–0.20	× 10^9/L
Metamyelocyte	3	%				
Myelocyte	3	%				
Band form	5	%				
NRBC	3 / 100 WBC					

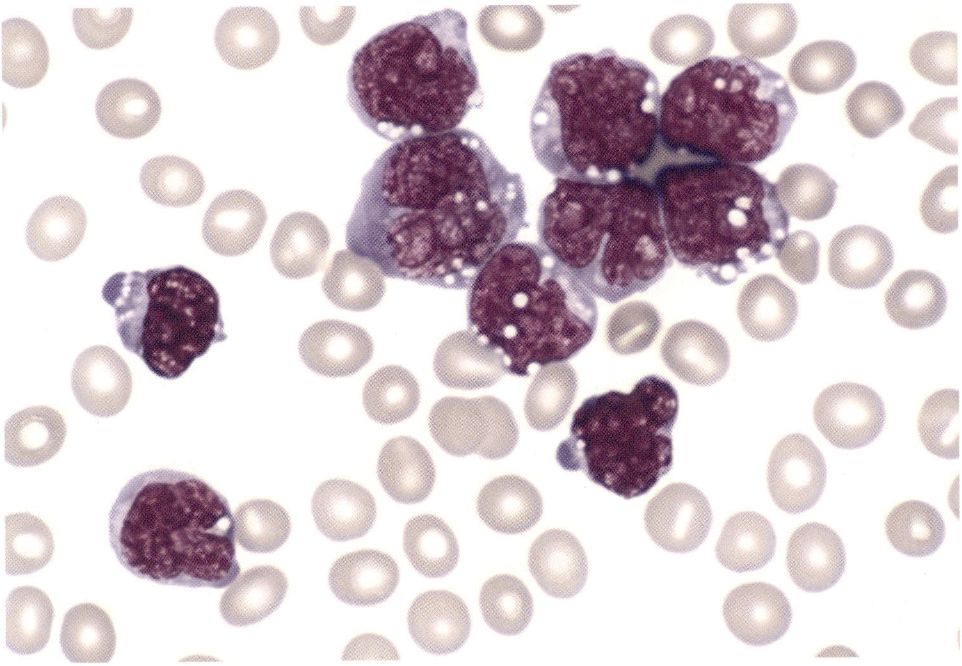

Blood film comments	
Red cell comments	Slight microcytes 3 NRBC / 100 WBC
White blood cell comments	Left shift in the myeloid line A very occasional cell with a high N/C ratio is seen on the blood film Leucoerythroblastic blood film
Platelet comments	Thrombocytopenia

Question 1. What is the differential diagnosis?

Based on the differential diagnosis, the following tests should be requested	
Bone marrow, trephine, immunophenotyping and cytogenetics	
Bone marrow	The marrow is heavily infiltrated with lymphoblasts with round nuclei, prominent nucleoli, intensely basophilic cytoplasm and prominent vacuolation. These lymphoblasts clearly resemble those of Burkitt cell leukaemia. Bone marrow trephine as above.
Immunophenotype	SIg^+, TdT^-, $HLA\text{-}DR^-$, $CD10^+$, $CD19^+$, $CD20^+$, $CD22^+$, $BCL6^+$, $CD38^+$, $CD77^+$, $CD43^+$ and $CD34^-$
Cytogenetics	When a clonal abnormality is present: t(8;14)(q24;q32), t(8;22)(q24;q11), t(2;8)(p12;q24)

Question 2. Are further tests indicated as part of your final report? If so, which tests?

(a)	Epstein Barr NA IgG antibody	Positive
	Epstein Barr VCA IgG antibody	Positive
	Epstein Barr VCA IgM antibody	Negative
(b)	HTLV 1+2 antibody	Negative

CASE STUDY 57

Case history

An 80-year-old female presents with a suspected pathological fracture of the femur.

Analyser data

Parameters	Test Results		Reference Range	
RBC	2.31	$\times 10^{12}$/L	3.80–5.80	$\times 10^{12}$/L
Hb	74	g/L	115–165	g/L
HCT	0.217		0.37–0.47	
MCV	93.9	fL	80–100	fL
MCH	32.0	pg	26.5–33.0	pg
MCHC	341	g/L	310–360	g/L
RDW-SD	49.7	fL	38.0–48.0	fL
RDW-CV	15.3	%	12.0–14.5	%
RETIC CT				
RETIC ABS				
WBC	12.8	$\times 10^9$/L	3.5–11.0	$\times 10^9$/L
Plat	159	$\times 10^9$/L	150–400	$\times 10^9$/L

Differential

Parameters	Test Results				Reference Range	
Neutrophil	90.0	%	11.5	$\times 10^9$/L	1.7–7.0	$\times 10^9$/L
Lymphocyte	4.0	%	0.5	$\times 10^9$/L	1.5–4.0	$\times 10^9$/L
Monocyte	4.0	%	0.5	$\times 10^9$/L	0.1–0.8	$\times 10^9$/L
Eosinophil	0.0	%	0.00	$\times 10^9$/L	0.04–0.44	$\times 10^9$/L
Basophil	0.0	%	0.00	$\times 10^9$/L	0.00–0.20	$\times 10^9$/L
Plasma cell	2.0	%				
ESR	84 mm/h				<20 mm/h	

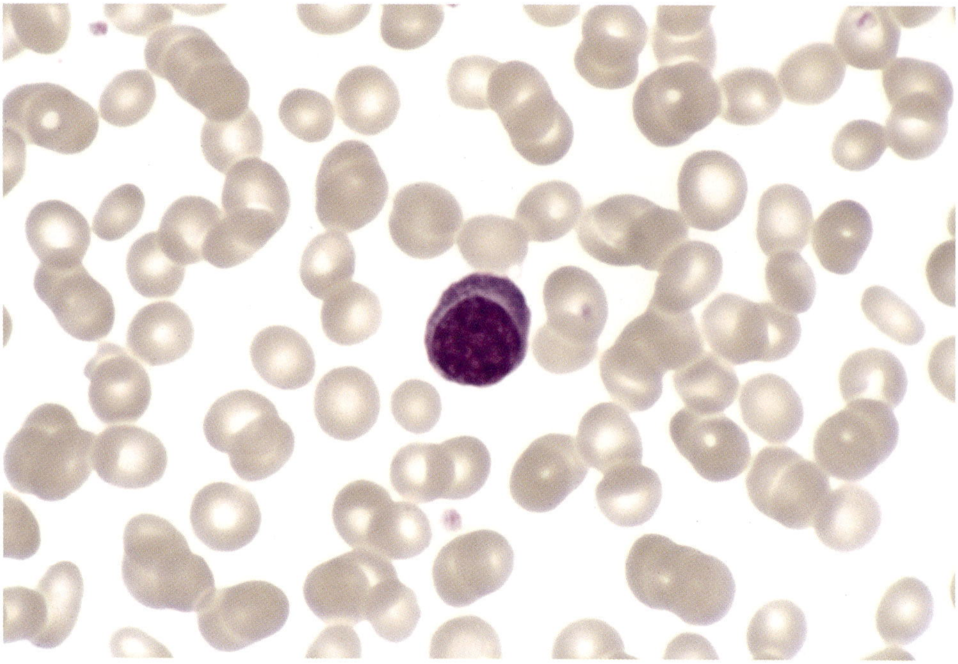

Blood film comments	
Red cell comments	Slight anisocytosis Moderate rouleaux
White blood cell comments	Neutrophilia Occasional circulating plasma cell
Platelet comments	Normal in number and morphology

Question 1. What is the differential diagnosis?

Based on the differential diagnosis, the following tests should be requested	
Bone marrow, trephine, immunophenotyping and cytogenetics	
Bone marrow	While the peripheral blood may contain few if any plasma cells, the bone marrow contains between 30% and 90% plasma cells. In severe cases there may be sheets of plasma cells. Binucleated plasma cells are also a common occurrence. Bone marrow trephine as above.
Immunophenotype	$CD19^-$, $CD20^-$, $CD138^+$, $CD38^+$, $CD56/58^+$, $CD79a^+$
Cytogenetics	Anomalies identified by FISH include: 1q abnormalities, t(11;14)(q13;q32), t(14;16)(q32;q23), t(4;14)(p16.3;q32), −13/del13q
A plasmacytoma is a solitary tumour of plasma cells identical to those that occur in plasma cell myeloma. Plasmacytomas occur in areas of active haemopoiesis such as the vertebrae, ribs and skull.	

Question 2. Are further tests indicated as part of your final report? If so, which tests?

Serum proteins				
Protein	74	g/L	RR (61–79)	g/L
Albumin	42	g/L	RR (33–48)	g/L
Alpha 1 Glob	1	g/L	RR (2.30–4.0)	g/L
Alpha 2 Glob	7	g/L	RR (5.0–9.0)	g/L
Beta Glob	17	g/L	RR (6.0–10.0)	g/L
Gamma Glob	7	g/L	RR (7.0–13.0)	g/L
Paraprotein 1	3	g/L		

MMUNOFIX IGGK
IGGK Immunofixation identifies paraprotein as IgG kappa.
PP1 Paraprotein of 3 g/L in the beta globulin region.
Bence-Jones protein (BJP): Positive
Immunofixation identifies BJP as free lambda light chains.
BJP excretion = 5.10 g/24 hours.

CASE STUDY 58

Case history

A 5-year-old child presents with easy bruising and lymphadenopathy.

Analyser data

Parameters	Test Results		Reference Range	
RBC	2.61	$\times 10^{12}/L$	3.96–4.92	$\times 10^{12}/L$
Hb	73	g/L	110–139	g/L
HCT	0.205		0.32–0.39	
MCV	78.5	fL	74–86	fL
MCH	28.0	pg	25.5–30.6	pg
MCHC	356	g/L	310–360	g/L
RDW-SD	42.9	fL	34.6–42.7	fL
RDW-CV	15.1	%	11.9–14.9	%
RETIC CT				
RETIC ABS				
WBC	25.0	$\times 10^9/L$	4.7–12.3	$\times 10^9/L$
Plat	78	$\times 10^9/L$	205–457	$\times 10^9/L$

Differential

Parameters	Test Results				Reference Range	
Neutrophil	2.0	%	0.5	$\times 10^9/L$	1.8–7.7	$\times 10^9/L$
Lymphocyte	16.0	%	4.0	$\times 10^9/L$	1.6–5.1	$\times 10^9/L$
Monocyte	0.0	%	0.0	$\times 10^9/L$	0.1–1.0	$\times 10^9/L$
Eosinophil	0.0	%	0.00	$\times 10^9/L$	0.0–0.6	$\times 10^9/L$
Basophil	0.0	%	0.00	$\times 10^9/L$	0.00–0.10	$\times 10^9/L$
Blast	82	%				

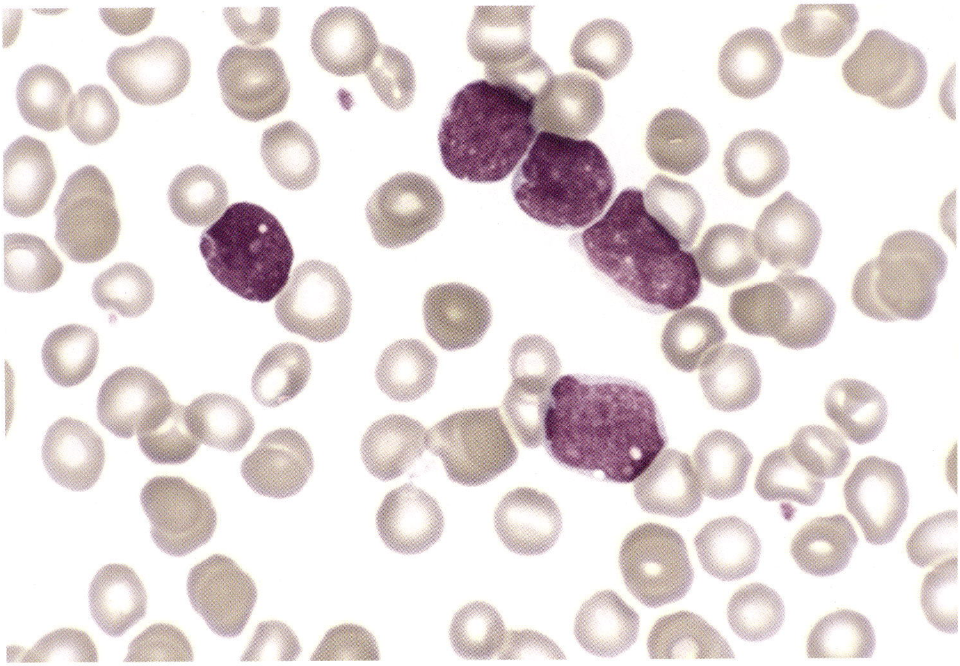

Blood film comments	
Red cell comments	Slight anisocytosis
White blood cell comments	82% blasts
Platelet comments	Thrombocytopenia

Question 1. What is the differential diagnosis?

Based on the differential diagnosis, the following tests should be requested	
Bone marrow, trephine, immunophenotyping and cytogenetics	
Bone marrow	The marrow is heavily infiltrated with a population of blast cells with a condensed nuclear chromatin pattern, inconspicuous nucleoli and a fine rim of basophilic cytoplasm. There are some larger blast cells present with more prominent nucleoli. Some of the blasts have vacuolated cytoplasm. Bone marrow trephine as above.
Immunophenotype	TdT^{+}, HLA-DR^{+}, SIg^{-}, cyt-μ^{-}-, $CD10^{+}$, $CD19^{+}$, $CD22^{-}$, $CD34^{+}$
Cytogenetics	t(12;21)(p13;q22), t(1;19)(q23;p13.3), t(9;22)(q34;q11.2), t(4;11)(q21;q23)

Question 2. Are further tests indicated as part of your final report? If so, which tests?

CASE STUDY 59

Case history

A 5-year-old child presents with a large mediastinal mass and difficulty with breathing.

Analyser data				
Parameters	**Test Results**		**Reference Range**	
RBC	3.86	$\times 10^{12}$/L	3.96–4.92	$\times 10^{12}$/L
Hb	102	g/L	110–139	g/L
HCT	0.308		0.32–0.39	
MCV	79.8	fL	74–86	fL
MCH	26.4	pg	25.5–30.6	pg
MCHC	331	g/L	310–360	g/L
RDW-SD	44.8	fL	34.6–42.7	fL
RDW-CV	15.5	%	11.9–14.9	%
RETIC CT				
RETIC ABS				
WBC	347.8	$\times 10^9$/L	4.7–12.3	$\times 10^9$/L
Plat	108	$\times 10^9$/L	205–457	$\times 10^9$/L

Differential						
Parameters	**Test Results**				**Reference Range**	
Neutrophil	4.0	%	13.9	$\times 10^9$/L	1.8–7.7	$\times 10^9$/L
Lymphocyte	4.0	%	13.9	$\times 10^9$/L	1.6–5.1	$\times 10^9$/L
Monocyte	1.0	%	3.48	$\times 10^9$/L	0.1–1.0	$\times 10^9$/L
Eosinophil	0.0	%	0.00	$\times 10^9$/L	0.0–0.6	$\times 10^9$/L
Basophil	0.0	%	0.00	$\times 10^9$/L	0.00–0.10	$\times 10^9$/L
Blast	91	%				

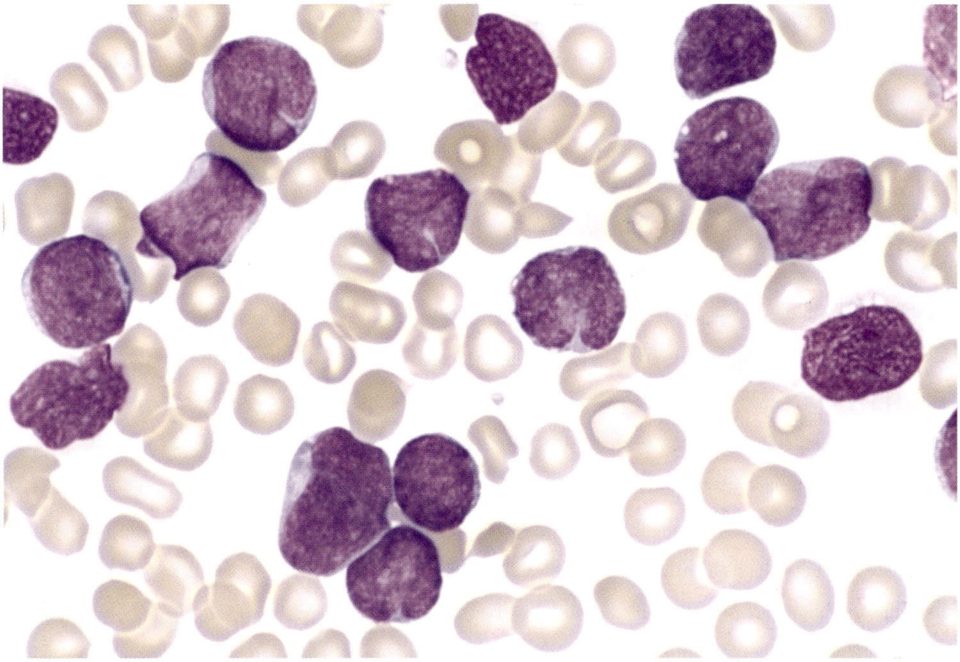

Blood film comments	
Red cell comments	Slight anisocytosis
White blood cell comments	91% blast cells
Platelet comments	Thrombocytopenia

Question 1. What is the differential diagnosis?

Based on the differential diagnosis, the following tests should be requested	
Bone marrow, trephine, immunophenotyping and cytogenetics	
Bone marrow	The marrow is heavily infiltrated with small to large blast cells. They have a condensed nuclear chromatin pattern, inconspicuous nucleoli and a fine rim of basophilic cytoplasm. Many of the blasts have folded, cleaved nuclei. Bone marrow trephine as above.
Immunophenotype	TdT^{+}, HLA-DR^{-}, CD1a^{+}, CD2^{+}, CD3^{+}, CD4$^{+/-}$, CD5^{+}, CD7^{+}, CD8$^{+/-}$
Cytogenetics	t(1;7)(p33;q34), t(7;9)(q34;q34), t(7;10)(q34;q24), t(7;11)(q34;p13), t(8;14)(q24;q11), t(10;14)(q24;q11), t(11;14)(p13;q11)

Question 2. Are further tests indicated as part of your final report? If so, which tests?

CASE STUDY 60

Case history

A 3-week-old febrile premature infant (31 weeks gestation).

Analyser data

Parameters	**Test Results**		**Reference Range**	
RBC	2.98	$\times 10^{12}$/L	3.38–3.94	$\times 10^{12}$/L
Hb	104	g/L	102–130	g/L
HCT	0.295		0.30–0.38	
MCV	98.0	fL	84–98	fL
MCH	34.9	pg	29.0–33.8	pg
MCHC	353	g/L	333–355	g/L
RDW-SD	57.6	fL	39.9–56.6	fL
RDW-CV	17.2	%	12.6–16.0	%
RETIC CT				
RETIC ABS				
WBC	28.3	$\times 10^9$/L	6.4–12.1	$\times 10^9$/L
Plat	83	$\times 10^9$/L	270–645	$\times 10^9$/L

Differential

Parameters	**Test Results**				**Reference Range**
Neutrophil	55.0	%	15.6	$\times 10^9$/L	0.8–4.9
Lymphocyte	6.0	%	1.7	$\times 10^9$/L	3.8–7.6
Monocyte	17.0	%	4.81	$\times 10^9$/L	0.3–1.2
Eosinophil	0.0	%	0.00	$\times 10^9$/L	0.10–0.80
Basophil	0.0	%	0.00	$\times 10^9$/L	0.00–0.20
Metamyelocyte	2	%			
Myelocyte	10	%			
Band form	10	%			
NRBC	2 / 100 WBC				

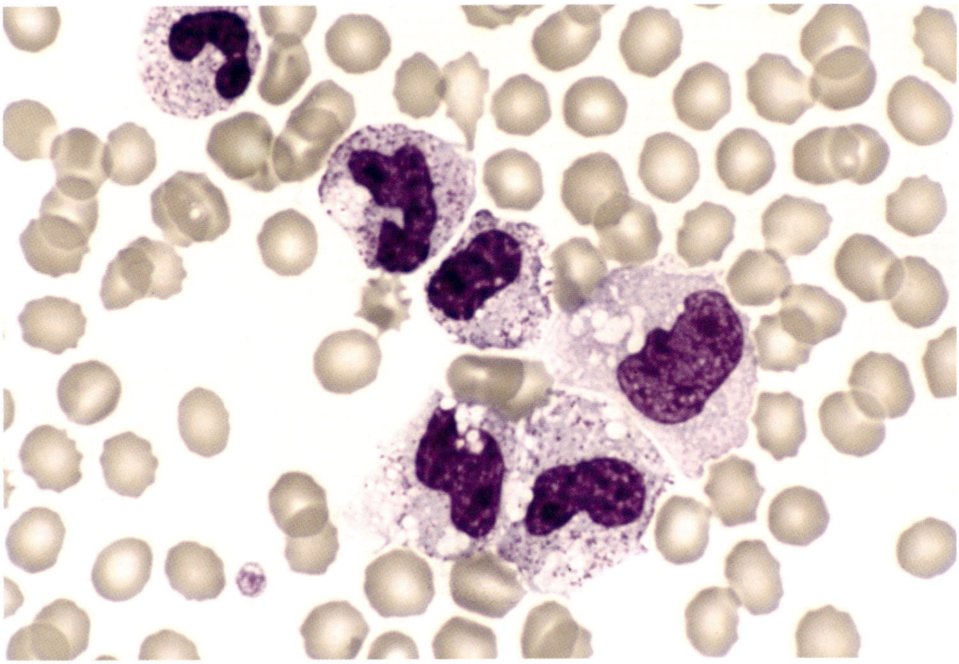

Blood film comments	
Red cell comments	Slight anisocytosis 2 NRBC / 100 WBC
White blood cell comments	Left shift in the myeloid line Moderate toxic granulation Moderate toxic vacuolation Neutrophilia Monocytosis
Platelet comments	Thrombocytopenia

Question 1. What is the differential diagnosis?

Based on the differential diagnosis, the following tests should be requested
The clinical history and the white cell count both point to a diagnosis of septicaemia. The importance of counting *every* myeloid precursor in a neonate cannot be overemphasised. Septicaemia is one of the most difficult decisions a neonatologist has to make, so the counting of every myeloid precursor is imperative. Septicaemia in a neonate has a high mortality rate. It is also important that the individual toxic changes be itemised rather than simply reporting slight, moderate or marked toxic changes.

Question 2. Are further tests indicated as part of your final report? If so, which tests?

CASE STUDY 61

Case history

A 6-month-old infant receiving chemotherapy for neuroblastoma.

Analyser data

Parameters	Test Results		Reference Range	
RBC	3.54	$\times 10^{12}$/L	3.88–5.13	$\times 10^{12}$/L
Hb	100	g/L	104–132	g/L
HCT	0.297		0.30–0.38	
MCV	83.0	fL	70–83	fL
MCH	28.2	pg	23.1–29.4	pg
MCHC	337	g/L	310–360	g/L
RDW-SD	47.1	fL	34.8–44.6	fL
RDW-CV	15.9	%	12.3–17.0	%
RETIC CT				
RETIC ABS				
WBC	38.6	$\times 10^9$/L	5.4–13.6	$\times 10^9$/L
Plat	69	$\times 10^9$/L	205–553	$\times 10^9$/L

Differential

Parameters	Test Results				Reference Range	
Neutrophil	72	%	27.8	$\times 10^9$/L	1.1–6.0	$\times 10^9$/L
Lymphocyte	5.0	%	1.9	$\times 10^9$/L	2.7–8.9	$\times 10^9$/L
Monocyte	11.0	%	4.2	$\times 10^9$/L	0.2–1.1	$\times 10^9$/L
Eosinophil	0.0	%	0.00	$\times 10^9$/L	0.00–0.60	$\times 10^9$/L
Basophil	0.0	%	0.00	$\times 10^9$/L	0.00–0.10	$\times 10^9$/L
Blast	1.0	%				
Myelocyte	5	%				
Band form	6	%				

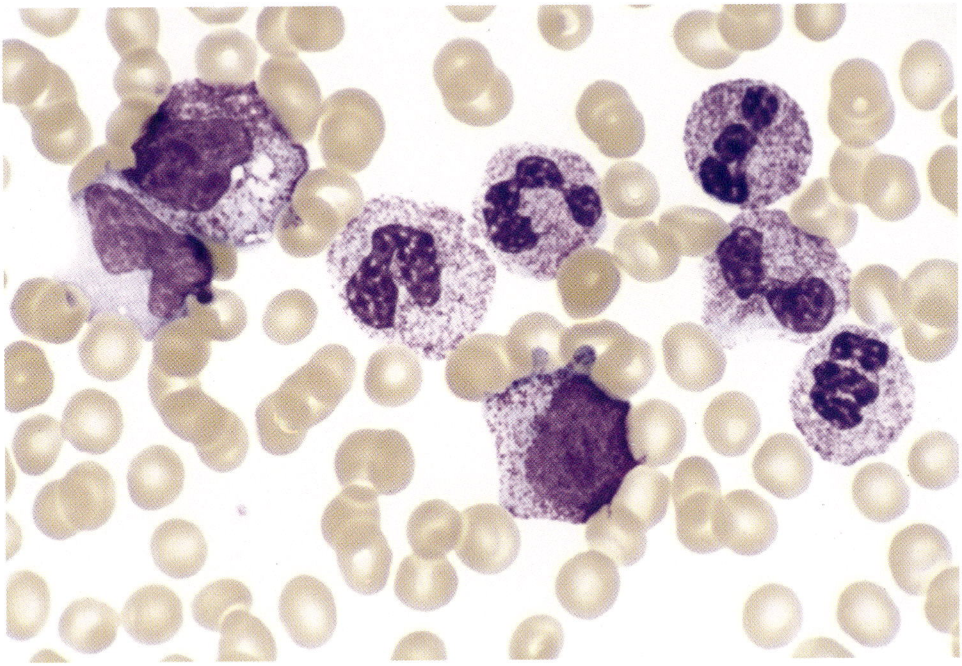

Blood film comments	
Red cell comments	Slight anisocytosis
White blood cell comments	Left shift in myeloid line Neutrophilia Increased neutrophil granulation ? on G-CSF therapy (granulocyte-colony stimulating factor)
Platelet comments	Thrombocytopenia

Question 1. What is the differential diagnosis?

Based on the differential diagnosis, the following tests should be requested
In this case study, full clinical notes are imperative. The fact that the child is having chemotherapy for neuroblastoma accounts for the thrombocytopenia, while the neutrophilia with a left shift suggests that the child is receiving cytokines, namely G-CSF. If this is the case and the child is receiving cytokine therapy, it would account for the increased neutrophil granulation, which is cytokine-induced rather than sepsis-induced.

Question 2. Are further tests indicated as part of your final report? If so, which tests?

CASE STUDY 62

Case history

A 1-year-old child presents with a persistent high fever for one week that is unresponsive to antibiotics.

Analyser data				
Parameters	**Test Results**		**Reference Range**	
RBC	3.49	$\times 10^{12}$/L	3.88–5.13	$\times 10^{12}$/L
Hb	89	g/L	104–132	g/L
HCT	0.265		0.30–0.38	
MCV	75.9	fL	70–83	fL
MCH	25.5	pg	23.1–29.4	pg
MCHC	336	g/L	310–360	g/L
RDW-SD	42.4	fL	34.8–44.6	fL
RDW-CV	13.2	%	12.3–17.0	%
RETIC CT				
RETIC ABS				
WBC	18.0	$\times 10^9$/L	5.4–13.6	$\times 10^9$/L
Plat	506	$\times 10^9$/L	205–553	$\times 10^9$/L
ESR	85 mm/h		<5 mm/h	

Differential						
Parameters	**Test Results**				**Reference Range**	
Neutrophil	66.5	%	11.9	$\times 10^9$/L	1.1–6.0	$\times 10^9$/L
Lymphocyte	26.2	%	4.7	$\times 10^9$/L	2.7–8.9	$\times 10^9$/L
Monocyte	3.3	%	0.6	$\times 10^9$/L	0.2–1.1	$\times 10^9$/L
Eosinophil	3.8	%	0.68	$\times 10^9$/L	0.00–0.60	$\times 10^9$/L
Basophil	0.2	%	0.03	$\times 10^9$/L	0.00–0.10	$\times 10^9$/L

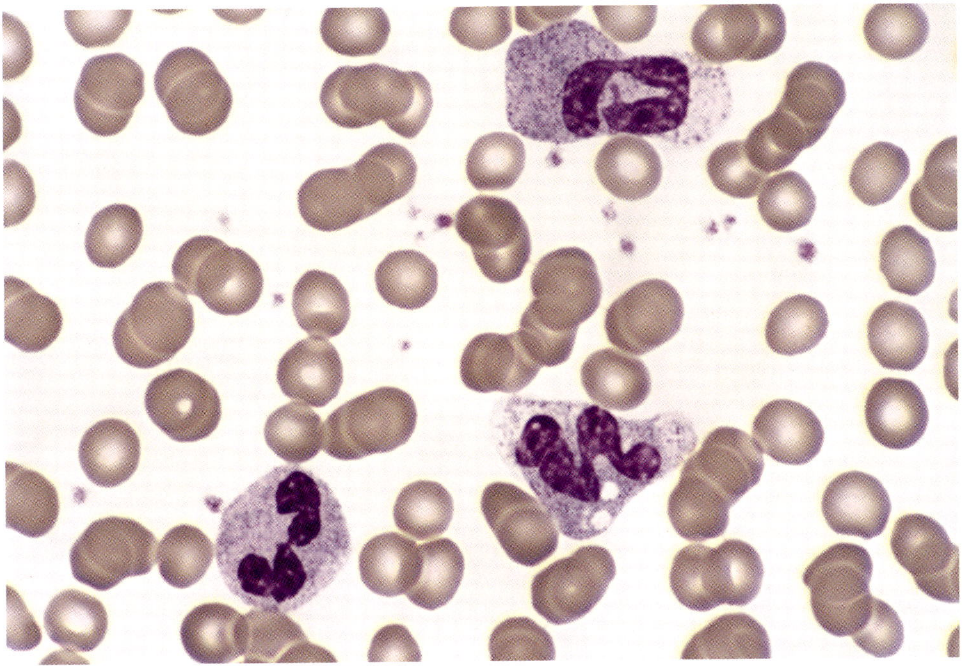

Blood film comments	
Red cell comments	Moderate rouleaux
White blood cell comments	Neutrophilia Moderate neutrophil granulation Slight vacuolation Neutrophils show cytoplasmic swelling, a feature seen in Kawasaki disease
Platelet comments	Normal in number and morphology

Question 1. What is the differential diagnosis?

Based on the differential diagnosis, the following tests should be requested
Septicaemia
Perform blood cultures. Check for growth / no growth. Septicaemia should respond to antibiotics.
Kawasaki disease
Kawasaki disease cannot be diagnosed by the blood film alone. Contact the paediatrician looking after the child and enquire as to the clinical features of the child. Kawasaki disease is characterised by the following: Non-exudative conjunctivitis; erythematous lips and a strawberry red tongue, erythematous and oedematous hands and feet and an erythematous truncal and desquamating perineal rash. The clinician will take the blood results and the clinical features of the child into consideration and make a diagnosis of Kawasaki disease if appropriate.

Question 2. Are further tests indicated as part of your final report? If so, which tests?

CASE STUDY 63

Case history

A 56-year-old male presents with bruising and bleeding gums.

Analyser data				
Parameters	**Test Results**		**Reference Range**	
RBC	2.92	$\times 10^{12}/L$	4.50–6.50	$\times 10^{12}/L$
Hb	95	g/L	130–180	g/L
HCT	0.271		0.40–0.54	
MCV	92.8	fL	80–100	fL
MCH	32.5	pg	26.5–33.0	pg
MCHC	351	g/L	310–360	g/L
RDW-SD	48.9	fL	38.0–48.0	fL
RDW-CV	14.7	%	12.0–14.5	%
RETIC CT				
RETIC ABS				
WBC	3.2	$\times 10^9/L$	3.5–11.0	$\times 10^9/L$
Plat	81	$\times 10^9/L$	150–400	$\times 10^9/L$

Differential						
Parameters	**Test Results**				**Reference Range**	
Neutrophil	23.0	%	0.7	$\times 10^9/L$	1.7–7.0	$\times 10^9/L$
Lymphocyte	28.0	%	0.9	$\times 10^9/L$	1.5–4.0	$\times 10^9/L$
Monocyte	3.0	%	0.10	$\times 10^9/L$	0.1–0.8	$\times 10^9/L$
Eosinophil	0.0	%	0.00	$\times 10^9/L$	0.04–0.44	$\times 10^9/L$
Basophil	0.0	%	0.00	$\times 10^9/L$	0.00–0.20	$\times 10^9/L$
Promyelocyte	17	%				
Metamyelocyte	6	%				
Myelocyte	23	%				

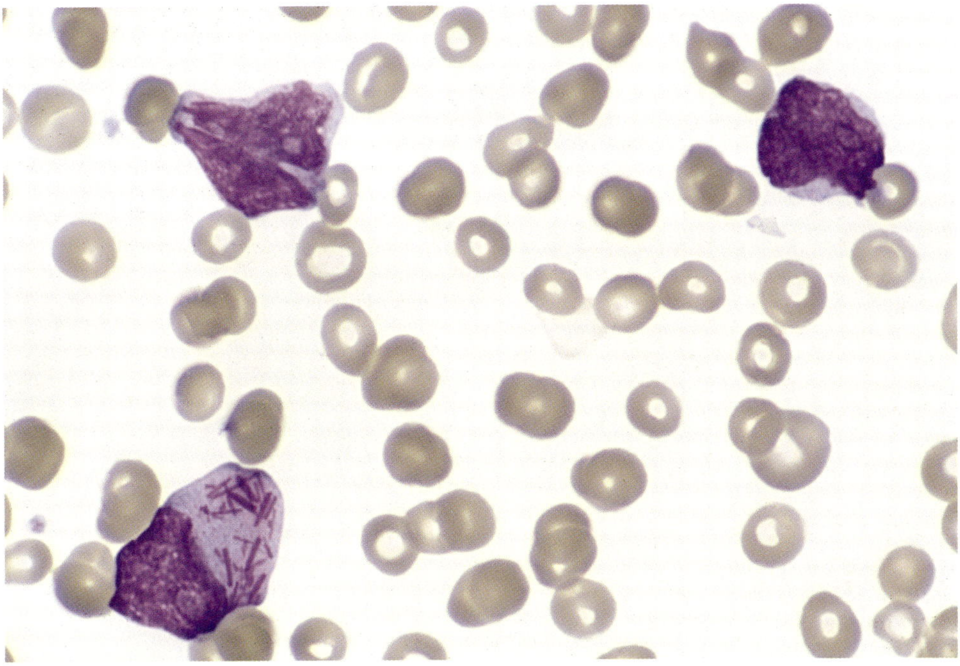

Blood film comments	
Red cell comments	Slight anisocytosis
White blood cell comments	Left shift in the myeloid line Neutropenia 17% abnormal promyelocytes Hypogranular, bilobed promyelocytes Auer rods and 'faggot' cells
Platelet comments	Thrombocytopenia

Question 1. What is the differential diagnosis?

Based on the differential diagnosis, the following tests should be requested	
Bone marrow, trephine, immunophenotyping and cytogenetics	
Bone marrow	The marrow is heavily infiltrated with promyelocytes whose nuclei vary in size and shape; many of them are bilobed and reniform shaped. Their cytoplasm is packed with large azurophilic granules. Many of the abnormal promyelocytes contain Auer rods and bundles of Auer rods or faggot cells. This is the hypergranular or typical type. Bone marrow trephine as above.
Immunophenotype	HLA-DR^{-}, CD13$^{+/-}$, CD33^{+}, CD117$^{-/+}$, CD34^{-}
Cytogenetics	t(15;17)(q22;q12)

Question 2. Are further tests indicated as part of your final report? If so, which tests?

Coagulation studies				
PT	13.6	sec	RR (12.0–15.0)	sec
IRR	1.0		RR (0.8–1.1)	
APTT	28.7	sec	RR (25.0–35.0)	sec
Fibrinogen	2.0	g/L	RR (2.20–4.30)	g/L
D-DIM LIA	9.65	μg/mL	RR (<0.5)	μg/mL
The above case has DIC. This is a medical emergency. A haematologist must be informed immediately.				

CASE STUDY 64

Case history

An 82-year-old female presents with lassitude and bruising.

Analyser data

Parameters	Test Results		Reference Range	
RBC	3.43	$\times 10^{12}$/L	3.80–5.80	$\times 10^{12}$/L
Hb	104	g/L	115–165	g/L
HCT	0.309		0.37–0.47	
MCV	90.1	fL	80–100	fL
MCH	30.3	pg	26.5–33.0	pg
MCHC	337	g/L	310–360	g/L
RDW-SD	50.1	fL	38.0–48.0	fL
RDW-CV	14.9	%	12.0–14.5	%
RETIC CT				
RETIC ABS				
WBC	4.02	$\times 10^9$/L	3.5–11.0	$\times 10^9$/L
Plat	99	$\times 10^9$/L	150–400	$\times 10^9$/L

Differential

Parameters	Test Results				Reference Range	
Neutrophil	55.0	%	2.2	$\times 10^9$/L	1.7–7.0	$\times 10^9$/L
Lymphocyte	3.0	%	0.1	$\times 10^9$/L	1.5–4.0	$\times 10^9$/L
Monocyte	2.0	%	0.1	$\times 10^9$/L	0.1–0.8	$\times 10^9$/L
Eosinophil	9.0	%	0.4	$\times 10^9$/L	0.04–0.44	$\times 10^9$/L
Basophil	0.0	%	0.00	$\times 10^9$/L	0.00–0.20	$\times 10^9$/L
Blast	28	%				
Myelocyte	1	%				
Band form	2	%				

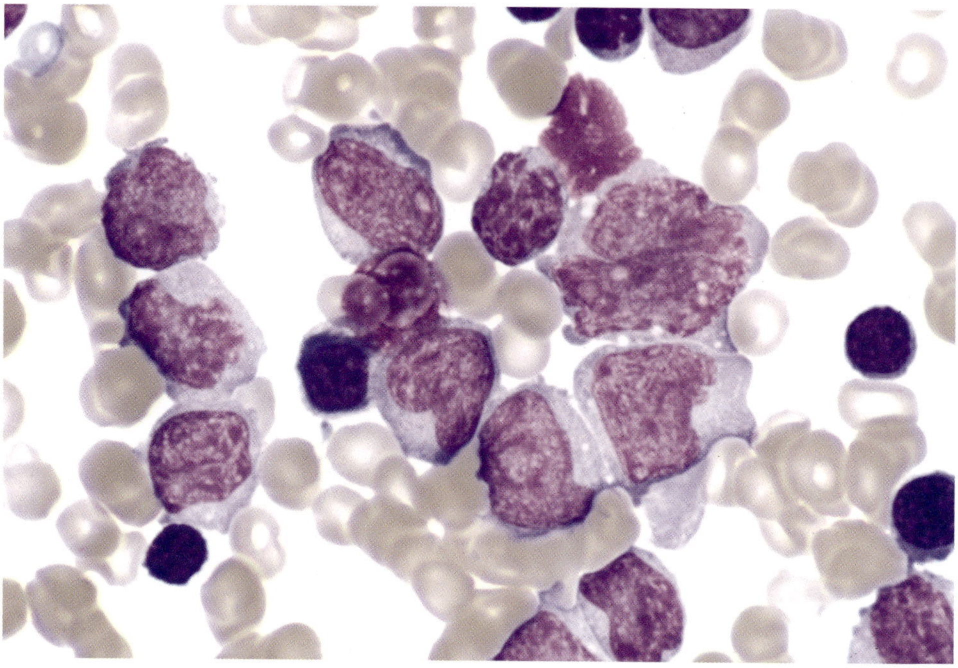

Blood film comments	
Red cell comments	Slight anisocytosis
White blood cell comments	Left shift in the myeloid line 28% blast cells
Platelet comments	Thrombocytopenia

Question 1. What is the differential diagnosis?

Based on the differential diagnosis, the following tests should be requested	
Bone marrow, trephine, immunophenotyping and cytogenetics	
Bone marrow	The blasts are medium sized with a high N/C ratio. The nuclei have a fine chromatin pattern with one to two clearly defined nucleoli and basophilic cytoplasm. They show no evidence of maturation. Bone marrow trephine as above.
Immunophenotype	HLA-DR⁺, CD13⁺, CD33⁺, CD38⁺, CD34⁺, CD117⁺
Cytogenetics	−5/del(5q)/rearrangements of 5, −7/del(7q)/rearrangements of 7, +8 and del(11q)

Question 2. Are further tests indicated as part of your final report? If so, which tests?

CASE STUDY 65

Case history
A 24-year-old male with bruising and petechiae.

Analyser data				
Parameters	**Test Results**		**Reference Range**	
RBC	2.78	$\times 10^{12}/L$	3.80–5.80	$\times 10^{12}/L$
Hb	84	g/L	115–165	g/L
HCT	0.246		0.37–0.47	
MCV	88.5	fL	80–100	fL
MCH	31.1	pg	26.5–33.0	pg
MCHC	30.2	g/L	310–360	g/L
RDW-SD	48.9	fL	38.0–48.0	fL
RDW-CV	15.7	%	12.0–14.5	%
RETIC CT				
RETIC ABS				
WBC	174.6	$\times 10^9/L$	3.5–11.0	$\times 10^9/L$
Plat	44	$\times 10^9/L$	150–400	$\times 10^9/L$

Differential						
Parameters	**Test Results**				**Reference Range**	
Neutrophil	10.0	%	17.5	$\times 10^9/L$	1.7–7.0	$\times 10^9/L$
Lymphocyte	2.0	%	3.5	$\times 10^9/L$	1.5–4.0	$\times 10^9/L$
Monocyte	5.0	%	8.73	$\times 10^9/L$	0.1–0.8	$\times 10^9/L$
Eosinophil	0.0	%	0.00	$\times 10^9/L$	0.04–0.44	$\times 10^9/L$
Basophil	0.0	%	0.00	$\times 10^9/L$	0.00–0.20	$\times 10^9/L$
Blast	83	%				

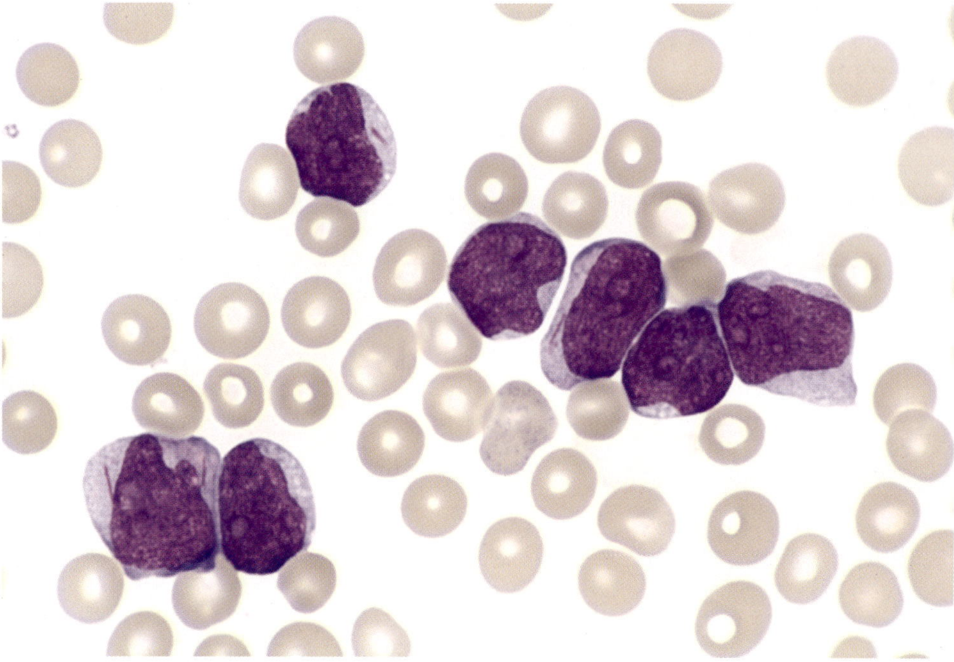

Blood film comments	
Red cell comments	Slight anisocytosis
White blood cell comments	83% blast cells Auer rods
Platelet comments	Thrombocytopenia

Question 1. What is the differential diagnosis?

Based on the differential diagnosis, the following tests should be requested	
Bone marrow, trephine, immunophenotyping and cytogenetics	
Bone marrow	The blasts have a high N/C ratio, round nuclei and fine chromatin pattern with one to two nucleoli. The cytoplasm is basophilic. Auer rods are present. Bone marrow trephine as above.
Immunophenotype	HLA-DR$^{+/-}$, CD13^{+}, CD33^{+}, CD34$^{+/-}$, CD117^{+}, CD15^{-}
Cytogenetics	No abnormality detected. No specific chromosomal abnormality is associated with this myeloid leukaemia.

Question 2. Are further tests indicated as part of your final report? If so, which tests?

CASE STUDY 66

Case history

A 69-year-old female presents with petechial rash.

Analyser data				
Parameters	**Test Results**		**Reference Range**	
RBC	3.89	$\times 10^{12}$/L	3.80–5.80	$\times 10^{12}$/L
Hb	111	g/L	115–165	g/L
HCT	0.337		0.37–0.47	
MCV	86.6	fL	80–100	fL
MCH	28.5	pg	26.5–33.0	pg
MCHC	329	g/L	310–360	g/L
RDW-SD	50.1	fL	38.0–48.0	fL
RDW-CV	15.2	%	12.0–14.5	%
RETIC CT				
RETIC ABS				
WBC	144.1	$\times 10^9$/L	3.5–11.0	$\times 10^9$/L
Plat	23	$\times 10^9$/L	150–400	$\times 10^9$/L

Differential						
Parameters	**Test Results**				**Reference Range**	
Neutrophil	4.0	%	5.8	$\times 10^9$/L	1.7–7.0	$\times 10^9$/L
Lymphocyte	17.0	%	24.5	$\times 10^9$/L	1.5–4.0	$\times 10^9$/L
Monocyte	3.0	%	4.32	$\times 10^9$/L	0.1–0.8	$\times 10^9$/L
Eosinophil	0.0	%	0.00	$\times 10^9$/L	0.04–0.44	$\times 10^9$/L
Basophil	0.0	%	0.00	$\times 10^9$/L	0.00–0.20	$\times 10^9$/L
Blast	57	%				
Promyelocyte	15	%				
Metamyelocyte	1	%				
Myelocyte	3	%				

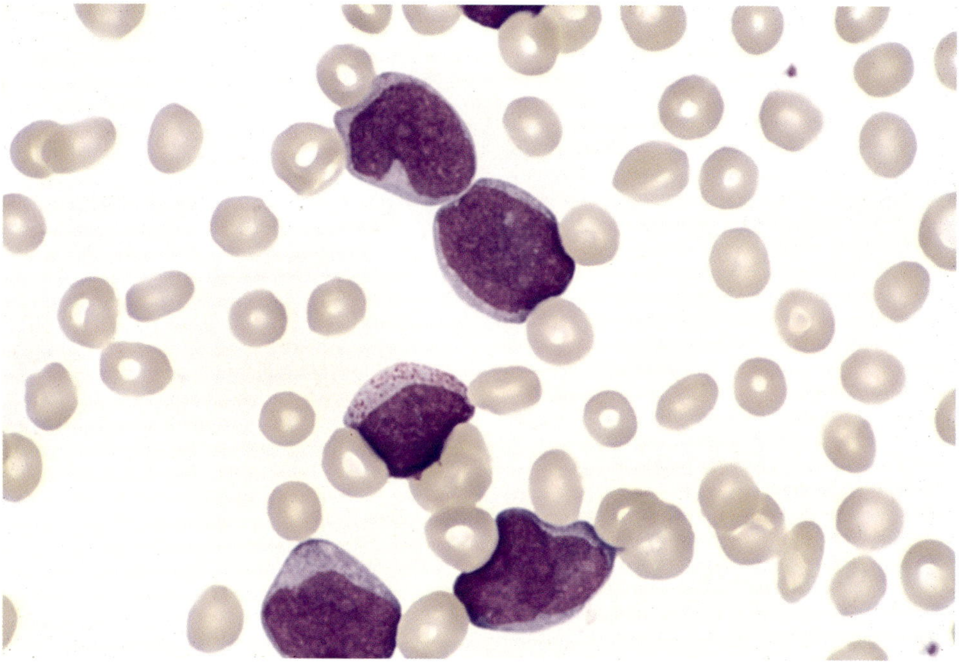

Blood film comments	
Red cell comments	Slight anisocytosis
White blood cell comments	Left shift in the myeloid line 57% blasts
Platelet comments	Thrombocytopenia

Question 1. What is the differential diagnosis?

Based on the differential diagnosis, the following tests should be requested	
Bone marrow, trephine, immunophenotyping and cytogenetics	
Bone marrow	The blasts have a high N/C ratio, round nuclei with nucleoli, varying amounts of cytoplasm with and without azurophilic granulation. Auer rods may be present. Promyelocytes, myelocytes and neutrophils make up at least 10% of the bone marrow cells. Bone marrow trephine as above.
Immunophenotype	HLA-DR$^{-/+}$, CD13^{+}, CD11b^{+}, CD15^{+}, CD33^{+}, CD34$^{-/+}$, CD117$^{-/+}$
Cytogenetics	No abnormality detected. No specific chromosomal abnormality is associated with this myeloid leukaemia.

Question 2. Are further tests indicated as part of your final report? If so, which tests?

CASE STUDY 67

Case history

A 59-year-old female presents with fever, fatigue and bruising.

Analyser data				
Parameters	**Test Results**		**Reference Range**	
RBC	2.38	× 10^{12}/L	3.80–5.80	× 10^{12}/L
Hb	76	g/L	115–165	g/L
HCT	0.239		0.37–0.47	
MCV	100.4	fL	80–100	fL
MCH	31.9	pg	26.5–33.0	pg
MCHC	318	g/L	310–360	g/L
RDW-SD	48.7	fL	38.0–48.0	fL
RDW-CV	14.9	%	12.0–14.5	%
RETIC CT	6.4	%	0.2–2.0	%
RETIC ABS	152.3	× 10^9/L	20–80	× 10^9/L
WBC	139.6	× 10^9/L	3.5–11.0	× 10^9/L
Plat	19	× 10^9/L	150–400	× 10^9/L

Differential						
Parameters	**Test Results**				**Reference Range**	
Neutrophil	20.0	%	2.8	× 10^9/L	1.7–7.0	× 10^9/L
Lymphocyte	4.0	%	5.6	× 10^9/L	1.5–4.0	× 10^9/L
Monocyte	68.0	%	94.9	× 10^9/L	0.1–0.8	× 10^9/L
Eosinophil	0.0	%	0.00	× 10^9/L	0.04–0.44	× 10^9/L
Basophil	0.0	%	0.00	× 10^9/L	0.00–0.20	× 10^9/L
Blast	24	%				
Metamyelocyte	1	%				
Myelocyte	1	%				

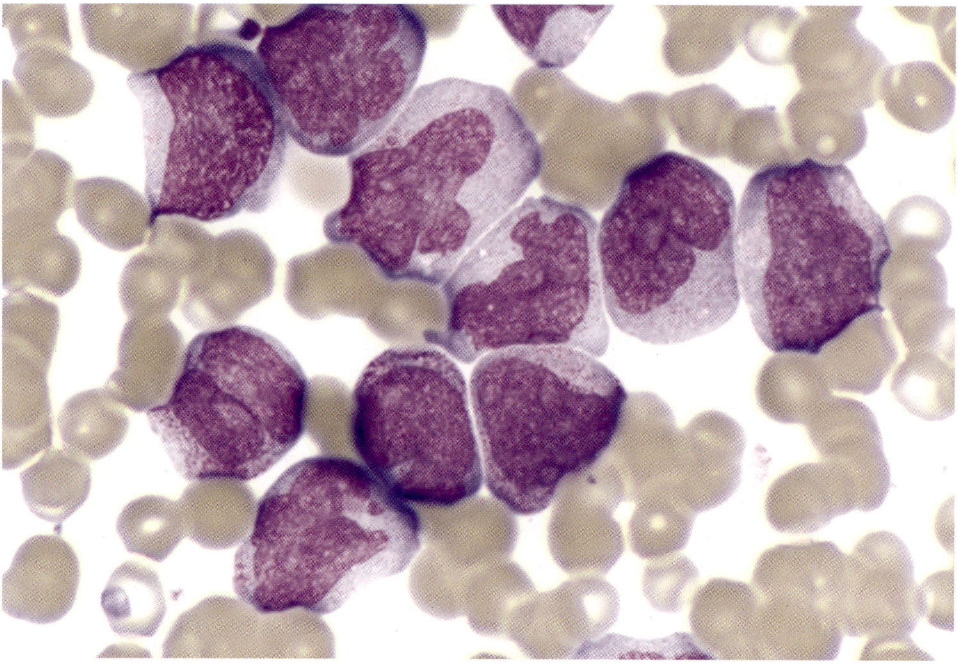

Blood film comments	
Red cell comments	Slight anisocytosis Moderate polychromasia
White blood cell comments	Left shift in the myeloid line Monocytosis 24% blast cells
Platelet comments	Thrombocytopenia

Question 1. What is the differential diagnosis?

Based on the differential diagnosis, the following tests should be requested	
Bone marrow, trephine, immunophenotyping and cytogenetics	
Bone marrow	The marrow is infiltrated with both myeloid precursors and myeloblasts as well as monocytes and monoblasts, including promonocytes. The myeloblasts have a high N/C ratio, round nuclei, fine chromatin pattern with one to two nucleoli. The cytoplasm is basophilic. The monoblasts are large cells with round nuclei, fine chromatin pattern and one or more nucleoli. Their cytoplasm is basophilic and may contain fine azurophilic granules. Should Auer rods be present, they will be in myeloblasts and not monoblasts. The promonocytes have a slightly convoluted, folded nucleus as well as nucleoli. Their cytoplasm is less basophilic; with a well stained film the cytoplasm will be seen to contain many fine azurophilic granules. Bone marrow trephine as above.

Immunophenotype	$CD13^+$, $CD33^+$, $CD15^+$, $CD65^+$, $CD34^{+/-}$ (myeloid markers) $CD4^+$, $CD11b^+$, $CD11c^+$, $CD14^+$, $CD36^+$, $CD64^+$ (monocytoid markers)
Cytogenetics	+8 There are no specific cytogenetic abnormalities in acute myelomonocytic leukaemia.

Question 2. Are further tests indicated as part of your final report? If so, which tests?

CASE STUDY 68

Case history

A 66-year-old male presents with bleeding gums.

Analyser data				
Parameters	**Test Results**		**Reference Range**	
RBC	3.29	× 10^{12}/L	4.50–6.50	× 10^{12}/L
Hb	112	g/L	130–180	g/L
HCT	0.339		0.40–0.54	
MCV	103.0	fL	80–100	fL
MCH	34.0	pg	26.5–33.0	pg
MCHC	330	g/L	310–360	g/L
RDW-SD	49.7	fL	38.0–48.0	fL
RDW-CV	15.6	%	12.0–14.5	%
RETIC CT				
RETIC ABS				
WBC	85.5	× 10^9/L	3.5–11.0	× 10^9/L
Plat	67	× 10^9/L	150–400	× 10^9/L

Differential						
Parameters	**Test Results**				**Reference Range**	
Neutrophil	1.0	%	0.9	× 10^9/L	1.7–7.0	× 10^9/L
Lymphocyte	2.0	%	1.7	× 10^9/L	1.5–4.0	× 10^9/L
Monocyte	1.0	%	0.9	× 10^9/L	0.1–0.8	× 10^9/L
Eosinophil	0.0	%	0.00	× 10^9/L	0.04–0.44	× 10^9/L
Basophil	0.0	%	0.00	× 10^9/L	0.00–0.20	× 10^9/L
Blast	96	%				

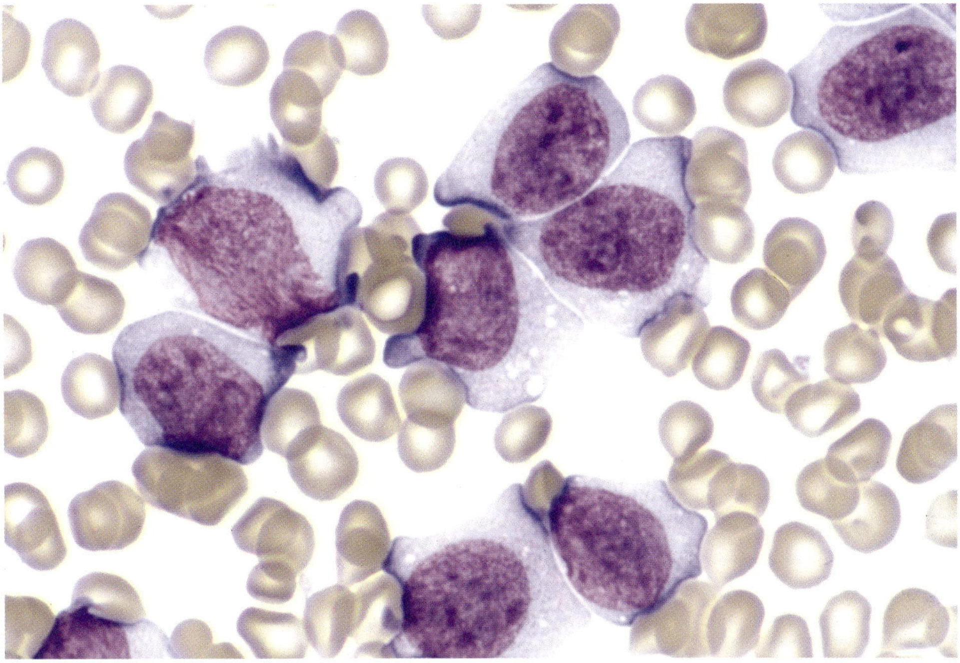

Blood film comments	
Red cell comments	Slight anisocytosis
White blood cell comments	96% blasts
Platelet comments	Thrombocytopenia

Question 1. What is the differential diagnosis?

Based on the differential diagnosis, the following tests should be requested	
Bone marrow, trephine, immunophenotyping and cytogenetics	
Bone marrow	The marrow is densely packed with monoblasts. The monoblasts are large cells with round nuclei, fine chromatin pattern and one or more nucleoli. Their cytoplasm is basophilic and may contain fine azurophilic granules. Bone marrow trephine as above.
Immunophenotype	$CD13^+$, $CD33^+$, $CD15^+$, $CD65^+$, $CD34^-$, $CD117^+$ (myeloid markers) $CD4^+$, $CD11b^+$, $CD11c^+$, $CD14^+$, $CD36^+$, $CD64^+$ $CD68^+$ (monocytoid markers)
Cytogenetics	t(8;16)(p11.2;p13.3)

Question 2. Are further tests indicated as part of your final report? If so, which tests?

CASE STUDY 69

Case history

A 56-year-old male with a past history of HIV-related non-Hodgkin lymphoma 5 years ago presents with anaemia and thrombocytopenia.

Analyser data

Parameters	Test Results		Reference Range	
RBC	3.20	× 10^{12}/L	4.50–6.50	× 10^{12}/L
Hb	99	g/L	130–180	g/L
HCT	0.298		0.40–0.54	
MCV	93.1	fL	80–100	fL
MCH	30.9	pg	26.5–33.0	pg
MCHC	332	g/L	310–360	g/L
RDW-SD	53.6	fL	38.0–48.0	fL
RDW-CV	16.4	%	12.0–14.5	%
RETIC CT				
RETIC ABS				
WBC	1.7	× 10^9/L	3.5–11.0	× 10^9/L
Plat	63	× 10^9/L	150–400	× 10^9/L
NRBC	23 / 100 WBC			

Differential

Parameters	Test Results				Reference Range	
Neutrophil	24.0	%	0.4	× 10^9/L	1.7–7.0	× 10^9/L
Lymphocyte	62.0	%	1.0	× 10^9/L	1.5–4.0	× 10^9/L
Monocyte	0.0	%	0.0	× 10^9/L	0.1–0.8	× 10^9/L
Eosinophil	0.0	%	0.00	× 10^9/L	0.04–0.44	× 10^9/L
Basophil	0.0	%	0.00	× 10^9/L	0.00–0.20	× 10^9/L
Blast	14	%				

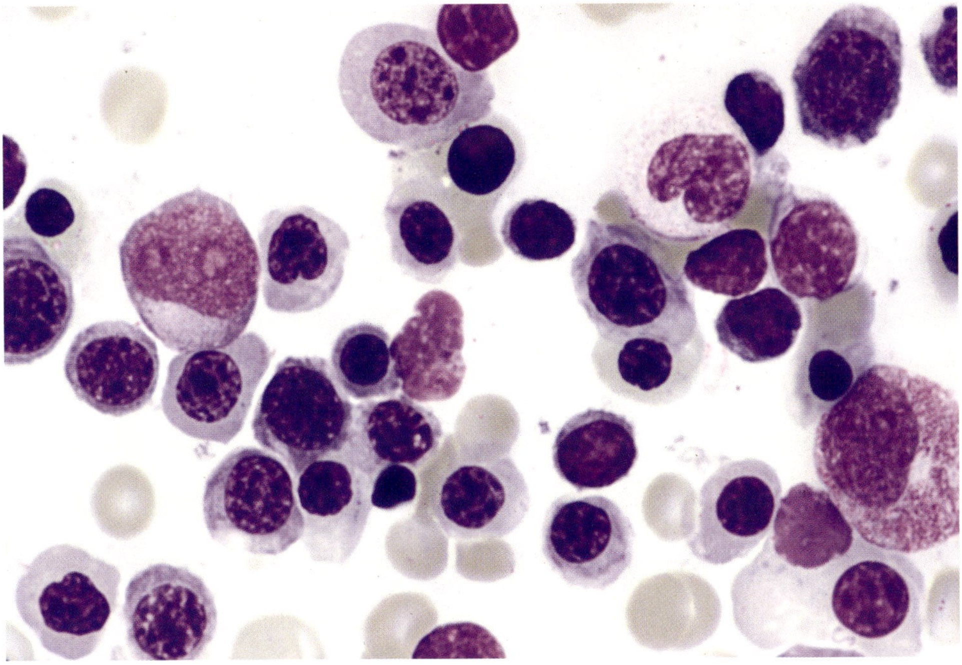

Blood film comments	
Red cell comments	Slight anisocytosis 23 NRBC / 100 WBC
White blood cell comments	14% blast cells
Platelet comments	Thrombocytopenia

Question 1. What is the differential diagnosis?

Based on the differential diagnosis, the following tests should be requested	
Bone marrow, trephine, immunophenotyping and cytogenetics	
Bone marrow	Erythropoiesis is markedly increased. All stages of maturation are represented, including proerythroblasts. The erythroblasts show marked dysplastic changes. Megaloblastoid forms with nuclear budding, binucleated and multinucleated nuclei. The cytoplasm is ragged with cytoplasmic blebbing and bridging. The myeloblasts have a high N/C ratio, round nuclei and fine chromatin pattern with one to two nucleoli. The cytoplasm is basophilic. In this case study, seventy per cent of the nucleated cells in the marrow are erythroid precursors and fifty-two per cent of the non-erythroid cells are myeloblasts. Bone marrow trephine as above.
Immunophenotype	HLA-DR$^{+/-}$, CD13^{+}, CD33^{+}, CD34$^{+/-}$, CD71$^{-/+}$
Cytogenetics	−5/del(5q), −7/del(7q), +8 No specific chromosomal abnormality; complex karyotypes are common.

Question 2. Are further tests indicated as part of your final report? If so, which tests?

CASE STUDY 70

Case history

A 2-year-old child presents with fever and bruising.

Analyser data				
Parameters	**Test Results**		**Reference Range**	
RBC	5.37	× 10^{12}/L	3.88–5.13	× 10^{12}/L
Hb	113	g/L	104–132	g/L
HCT	0.342		0.3–0.38	
MCV	95.0	fL	70–83	fL
MCH	31.3	pg	23.1–29.4	pg
MCHC	329	g/L	310–360	g/L
RDW-SD	37.2	fL	34.8–44.6	fL
RDW-CV	13.0	%	12.3–17.0	%
RETIC CT	3.1	%	0.2–2.0	%
RETIC ABS	166.5	× 10^9/L	20–80	× 10^9/L
WBC	5.4	× 10^9/L	5.4–13.6	× 10^9/L
Plat	18	× 10^9/L	205–553	× 10^9/L

Differential						
Parameters	**Test Results**				**Reference Range**	
Neutrophil	11.0	%	0.6	× 10^9/L	1.1–6.0	× 10^9/L
Lymphocyte	62.0	%	3.3	× 10^9/L	2.7–8.9	× 10^9/L
Monocyte	4.0	%	0.2	× 10^9/L	0.2–1.1	× 10^9/L
Eosinophil	0.0	%	0.00	× 10^9/L	0.00–0.60	× 10^9/L
Basophil	0.0	%	0.00	× 10^9/L	0.00–0.10	× 10^9/L
Blast	23	%				

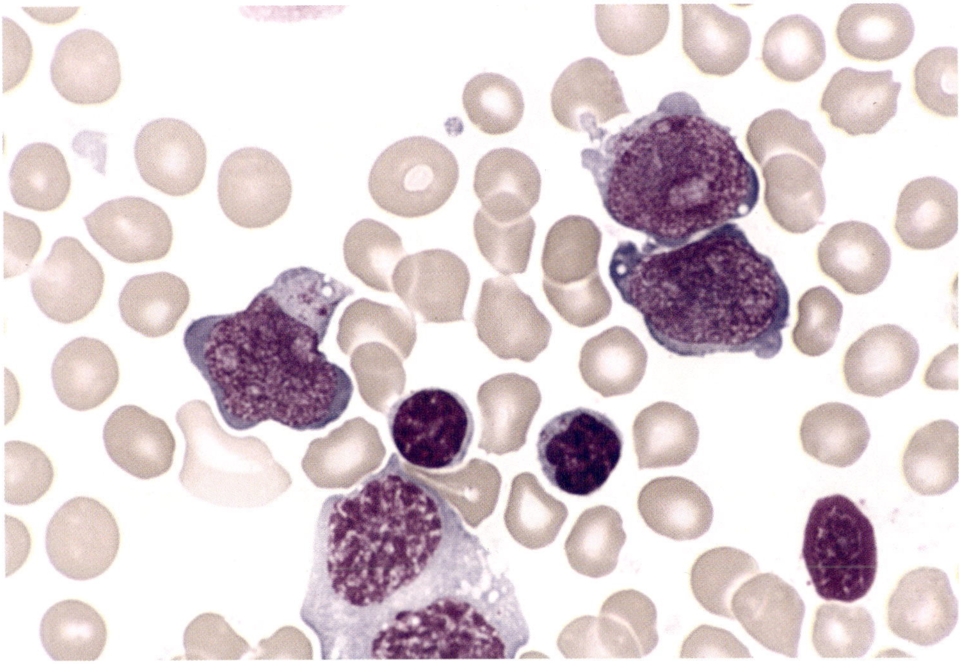

Blood film comments	
Red cell comments	Slight polychromasia
White blood cell comments	23% blast cells
Platelet comments	Thrombocytopenia

Question 1. What is the differential diagnosis?

Based on the differential diagnosis, the following tests should be requested	
Bone marrow, trephine, immunophenotyping and cytogenetics	
Bone marrow	Hypercellular marrow with dysplastic changes in all three cell lines. There is a heavy infiltrate of blast cells. The blasts are medium to large in size. They have a round nucleus with fine chromatin pattern and one to three nucleoli. The cytoplasm is basophilic with many of the blasts demonstrating cytoplasmic blebs and buds. The megakaryocytes are dysplastic; small megakaryoblasts are present. A reticulin stain on the marrow shows increased fibrosis. In many cases the increased fibrosis results in a dry tap when aspirating the bone marrow. Bone marrow trephine as above.
Immunophenotype	HLA-DR^{-}, CD13^{-}, CD33$^{+/-}$, CD34^{-}, CD41^{+}, CD45^{-}, CD61^{+}
Cytogenetics	inv(3)(q21;q26.2) and t(3;3)(q21;q26.2) There is no specific chromosomal abnormality.

Question 2. Are further tests indicated as part of your final report? If so, which tests?

CASE STUDY 71

Case history

A 10-day-old infant with Down syndrome (trisomy 21) transferred from another hospital.

Analyser data				
Parameters	**Test Results**		**Reference Range**	
RBC	3.74	$\times 10^{12}$/L	3.80–5.50	$\times 10^{12}$/L
Hb	130	g/L	120–185	g/L
HCT	0.370		0.36–0.55	
MCV	98.9	fL	95–100	fL
MCH	34.8	pg	31.5–33.6	pg
MCHC	351	g/L	310–360	g/L
RDW-SD	72.5	fL	50.0–70.0	fL
RDW-CV	26.6	%	12.0–18.0	%
RETIC CT				
RETIC ABS				
WBC	64.7	$\times 10^9$/L	6.8–20.0	$\times 10^9$/L
Plat	77	$\times 10^9$/L	250–600	$\times 10^9$/L

Differential						
Parameters	**Test Results**				**Reference Range**	
Neutrophil	13.0	%	8.4	$\times 10^9$/L	1.0–12.0	$\times 10^9$/L
Lymphocyte	37.0	%	24.0	$\times 10^9$/L	2.4–15.0	$\times 10^9$/L
Monocyte	4.0	%	2.6	$\times 10^9$/L	0.3–1.5	$\times 10^9$/L
Eosinophil	1.0	%	0.65	$\times 10^9$/L	0.10–1.30	$\times 10^9$/L
Basophil Blast	0.0 45	% %	0.00	$\times 10^9$/L	0.00–0.40	$\times 10^9$/L

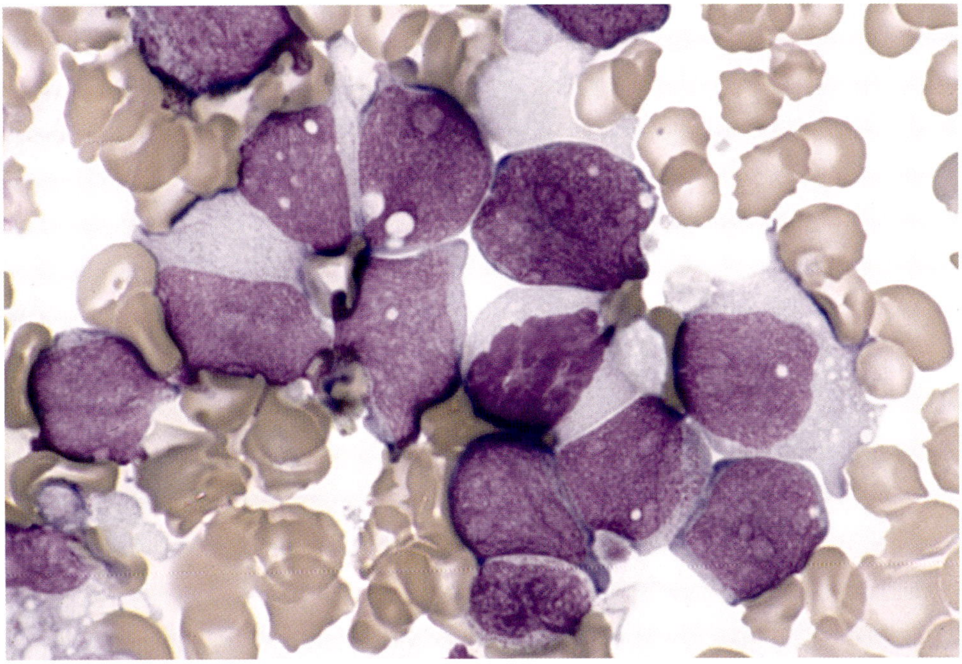

Blood film comments	
Red cell comments	Slight anisocytosis
White blood cell comments	45% blast cells
Platelet comments	Thrombocytopenia Large and giant platelets The mean platelet volume (MPV) and platelet distribution width (PDW) are increased.

Question 1. What is the differential diagnosis?

Based on the differential diagnosis, the following tests should be requested
Watch and wait!
Should this infant have TAM, the white cell count will spontaneously return to normal and the blasts will disappear. This will occur over a period of weeks (less than 3 months). Twenty-five per cent of infants with TAM will go on to develop megakaryoblastic leukaemia by the age of 3 years.
Should the infant have congenital leukaemia the white cell count will remain high and the blasts will persist. Treatment for acute leukaemia will commence.
Immunophenotyping may be performed on the peripheral blood. The markers expressed by TAM resemble those expressed by megakaryoblastic leukaemia, namely:
HLA-DR$^{-/+}$, CD34^{+}, CD117^{+}, CD13^{+}, CD33^{+}, CD7^{+}, CD45^{-}, CD41^{+}, CD61^{+}
In addition to the trisomy 21 of Down syndrome, no specific chromosomal abnormalities are associated with TAM.

Question 2. Are further tests indicated as part of your final report? If so, which tests?

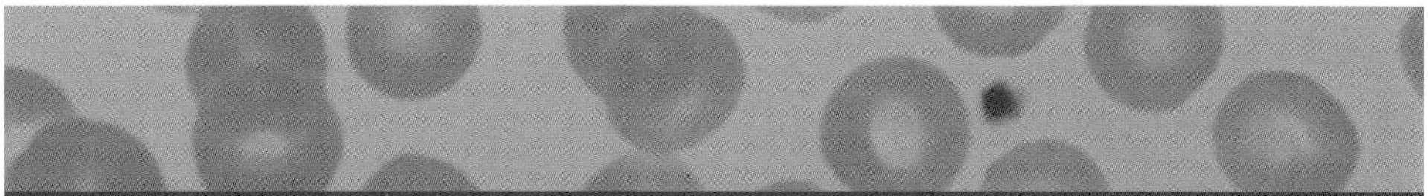

4
Platelet Cases

CASE STUDY 72

Case history

A 2-year-old child having a preoperative full blood count.

Analyser data				
Parameters	**Test Results**		**Reference Range**	
RBC	5.35	$\times 10^{12}$/L	3.88–5.13	$\times 10^{12}$/L
Hb	115	g/L	104–132	g/L
HCT	0.367		0.30–0.38	
MCV	68.6	fL	70–83	fL
MCH	21.5	pg	23.1–29.4	pg
MCHC	313	g/L	310–360	g/L
RDW-SD	35.7	fL	34.8–44.6	fL
RDW-CV	13.4	%	12.3–17.0	%
RETIC CT	2.3	%	0.2–2.0	%
RETIC ABS	123.0	$\times 10^9$/L	20–80	$\times 10^9$/L
WBC	10.9	$\times 10^9$/L	5.4–13.6	$\times 10^9$/L
Plat	133	$\times 10^9$/L	205–553	$\times 10^9$/L

Differential						
Parameters	**Test Results**				**Reference Range**	
Neutrophil	54.0	%	5.9	$\times 10^9$/L	1.7–7.0	$\times 10^9$/L
Lymphocyte	33.0	%	3.6	$\times 10^9$/L	1.5–4.0	$\times 10^9$/L
Monocyte	5.0	%	0.6	$\times 10^9$/L	0.1–0.8	$\times 10^9$/L
Eosinophil	6.0	%	0.7	$\times 10^9$/L	0.04–0.44	$\times 10^9$/L
Basophil	2.0	%	0.2	$\times 10^9$/L	0.00–0.20	$\times 10^9$/L

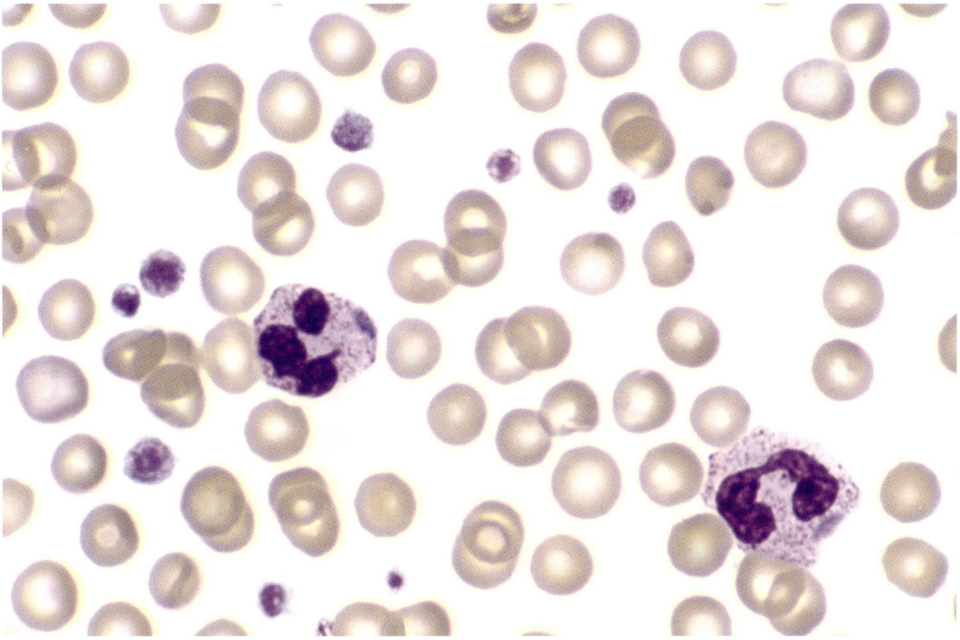

Blood film comments	
Red cell comments	Slight microcytes Slight hypochromasia It would be inappropriate to suggest iron studies on a 2-year-old child with the above MCV and MCH.
White blood cell comments	Slight eosinophilia Döhle bodies in the cytoplasm of otherwise normal neutrophils
Platelet comments	Thrombocytopenia Large platelets The mean platelet volume (MPV) and platelet distribution width (PDW) are increased. Process the blood through the optical mode of the blood cell analyser to ensure the large and giant platelets are included in the platelet count.

Question 1. What is the differential diagnosis?

Based on the differential diagnosis, the following tests should be requested					
MPV	13.6	fL	RR (7.4–11.5)	fL
PDW	17.2	fL	RR (12–15.6)	fL
Careful morphological examination of the blood film will differentiate between May-Hegglin anomaly and Bernard-Soulier syndrome. Both disorders are characterised by thrombocytopenia with large and giant platelets. The neutrophils of May-Hegglin anomaly contain Döhle bodies while the neutrophils in Bernard-Soulier syndrome are morphologically normal.				

Question 2. Are further tests indicated as part of your final report? If so, which tests?

CASE STUDY 73

Case history

A 4-year-old child with thrombocytopenia for investigation.

Analyser data				
Parameters	**Test Results**		**Reference Range**	
RBC	4.34	× 10^{12}/L	3.96–4.92	× 10^{12}/L
Hb	126	g/L	110–139	g/L
HCT	0.362		0.32–0.39	
MCV	83.4	fL	74–86	fL
MCH	29.0	pg	25.5–30.6	pg
MCHC	348	g/L	310–360	g/L
RDW-SD	35.2	fL	34.3–44.1	fL
RDW-CV	13.7	%	12.1–15.6	%
RETIC CT				
RETIC ABS				
WBC	9.2	× 10^9/L	4.7–12.3	× 10^9/L
Plat	69	× 10^9/L	205–457	× 10^9/L

Differential						
Parameters	**Test Results**				**Reference Range**	
Neutrophil	47.5	%	4.4	× 10^9/L	1.8–7.7	× 10^9/L
Lymphocyte	47.3	%	4.3	× 10^9/L	1.6–5.1	× 10^9/L
Monocyte	1.6	%	0.2	× 10^9/L	0.1–1.0	× 10^9/L
Eosinophil	3.1	%	0.3	× 10^9/L	0.00–0.60	× 10^9/L
Basophil	0.5	%	0.1	× 10^9/L	0.00–0.10	× 10^9/L

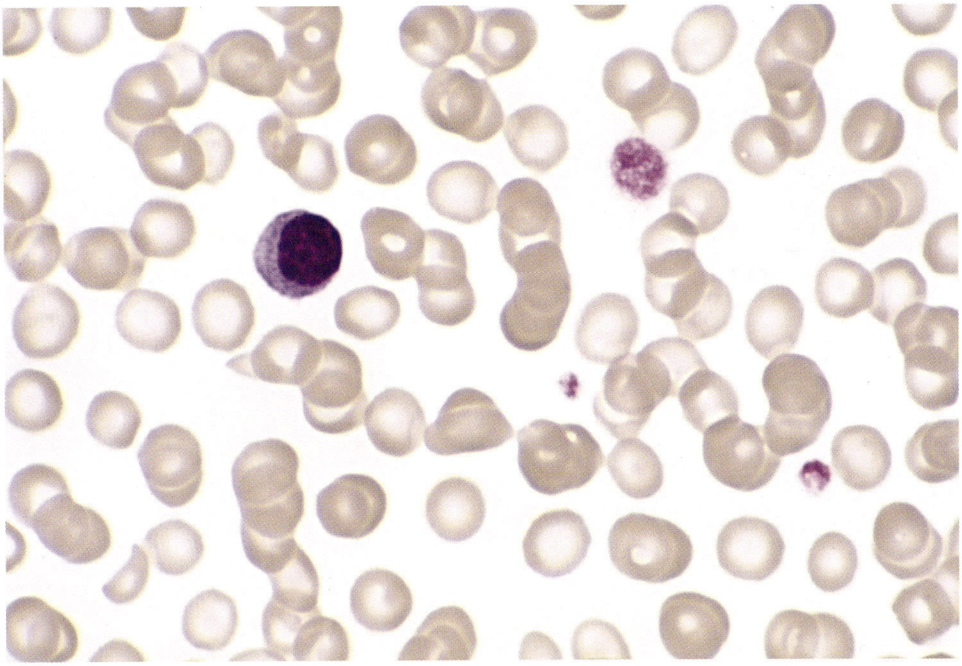

Blood film comments	
Red cell comments	Normal in number and morphology
White blood cell comments	Normal in number and morphology
Platelets comments	Thrombocytopenia Large and giant platelets The mean platelet volume (MPV) and platelet distribution width (PDW) are increased. Process the blood through the optical mode of the blood cell analyser to ensure the large and giant platelets are included in the platelet count.

Question 1. What is the differential diagnosis?

Based on the differential diagnosis, the following tests should be requested				
MPV	14.6	fL	RR (7.4–11.5)	fL
PDW	18.1	fL	RR (12–15.6)	fL

Careful morphological examination of the blood film shows morphologically normal neutrophils; there are no Döhle bodies.

To confirm Bernard-Soulier syndrome, platelet aggregation studies should be performed.

Platelet aggregation studies

Ristocetin	Absent aggregation
Arachidonic acid	Normal aggregation
Collagen	Normal aggregation

ADP	Normal aggregation
Adrenaline	Normal aggregation
Platelet aggregation results Platelet aggregation within normal limits for collagen, ADP, arachidonic acid and adrenaline. Absent platelet aggregation with ristocetin. Monoclonal antibody typing of platelet glycoprotein by flow cytometry shows reduced glycoprotein 1b-V-1X complex compared with the normal control. Results consistent with Bernard-Soulier syndrome.	

Question 2. Are further tests indicated as part of your final report? If so, which tests?

CASE STUDY 74

Case history

A 6-month-old child with thrombocytopenia for investigation.

Analyser data				
Parameters	**Test Results**		**Reference Range**	
RBC	4.12	× 10^{12}/L	3.39–4.86	× 10^{12}/L
Hb	112	g/L	100–122	g/L
HCT	0.345		0.28–0.36	
MCV	83.7	fL	68–85	fL
MCH	27.2	pg	22.6–29.7	pg
MCHC	325	g/L	310–360	g/L
RDW-SD	47.3	fL	34.0–42.4	fL
RDW-CV	15.4	%	12.0–14.8	%
RETIC CT				
RETIC ABS				
WBC	10.0	× 10^9/L	5.6–14.1	× 10^9/L
Plat	16	× 10^9/L	296–686	× 10^9/L

Differential						
Parameters	**Test Results**				**Reference Range**	
Neutrophil	68.4	%	6.8	× 10^9/L	0.5–4.4	× 10^9/L
Lymphocyte	17.1	%	1.7	× 10^9/L	3.4–9.8	× 10^9/L
Monocyte	9.7	%	1.0	× 10^9/L	0.2–1.0	× 10^9/L
Eosinophil	4.3	%	0.4	× 10^9/L	0.00–0.70	× 10^9/L
Basophil	0.5	%	0.1	× 10^9/L	0.00–0.10	× 10^9/L

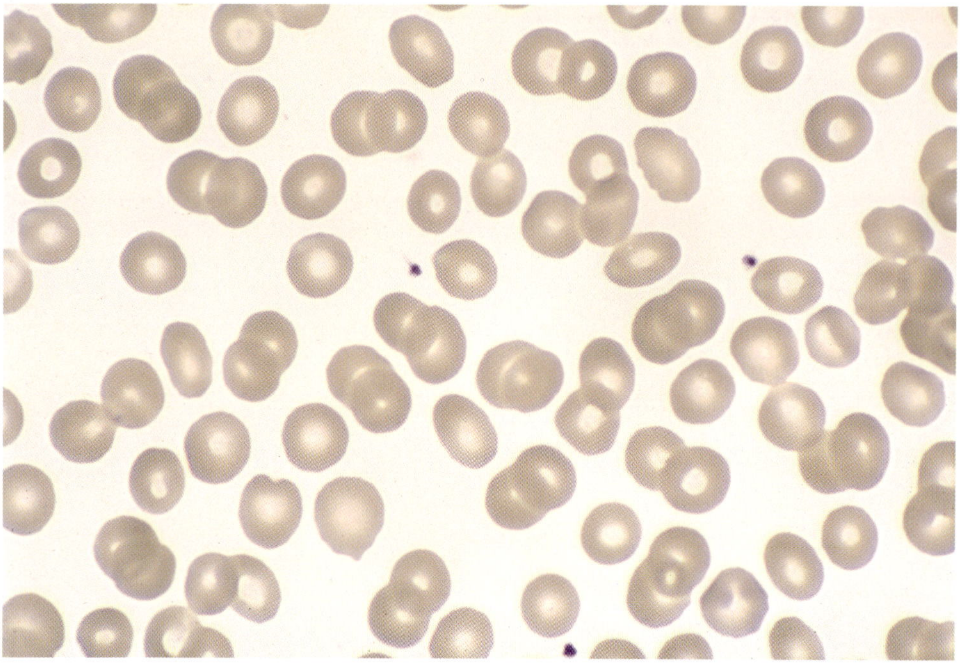

Blood film comments	
Red cell comments	Slight anisocytosis
White blood cell comments	Neutrophilia Lymphopenia
Platelet comments	Thrombocytopenia with small platelets The mean platelet volume (MPV) and platelet distribution width (PDW) are decreased.

Question 1. What is the differential diagnosis?

Based on the differential diagnosis, the following tests should be requested				
MPV	7.0	fL	RR (7.4–11.5)	fL
PDW	13	fL	RR (12–15.6)	fL
Bone marrow Normal to high numbers of megakaryocytes.				

Question 2. Are further tests indicated as part of your final report? If so, which tests?

CASE STUDY 75

Case history

An 18-month-old child presents with a petechial rash.

Analyser data				
Parameters	**Test Results**		**Reference Range**	
RBC	4.79	× 10^{12}/L	3.88–5.03	× 10^{12}/L
Hb	131	g/L	104–132	g/L
HCT	0.381		0.30–0.38	
MCV	79.5	fL	70–83	fL
MCH	27.3	pg	23.1–29.4	pg
MCHC	344	g/L	310–360	g/L
RDW-SD	35.6	fL	34.8–44.6	fL
RDW-CV	13.1	%	12.3–17.0	%
RETIC CT				
RETIC ABS				
WBC	18.4	× 10^9/L	5.4–13.6	× 10^9/L
Plat	3	× 10^9/L	205–553	× 10^9/L

Differential						
Parameters	**Test Results**				**Reference Range**	
Neutrophil	50.1	%	9.2	× 10^9/L	1.1–6.0	× 10^9/L
Lymphocyte	41.7	%	7.7	× 10^9/L	2.7–8.9	× 10^9/L
Monocyte	5.6	%	1.0	× 10^9/L	0.2–1.1	× 10^9/L
Eosinophil	2.3	%	0.4	× 10^9/L	0.00–0.60	× 10^9/L
Basophil	0.3	%	0.1	× 10^9/L	0.00–0.10	× 10^9/L

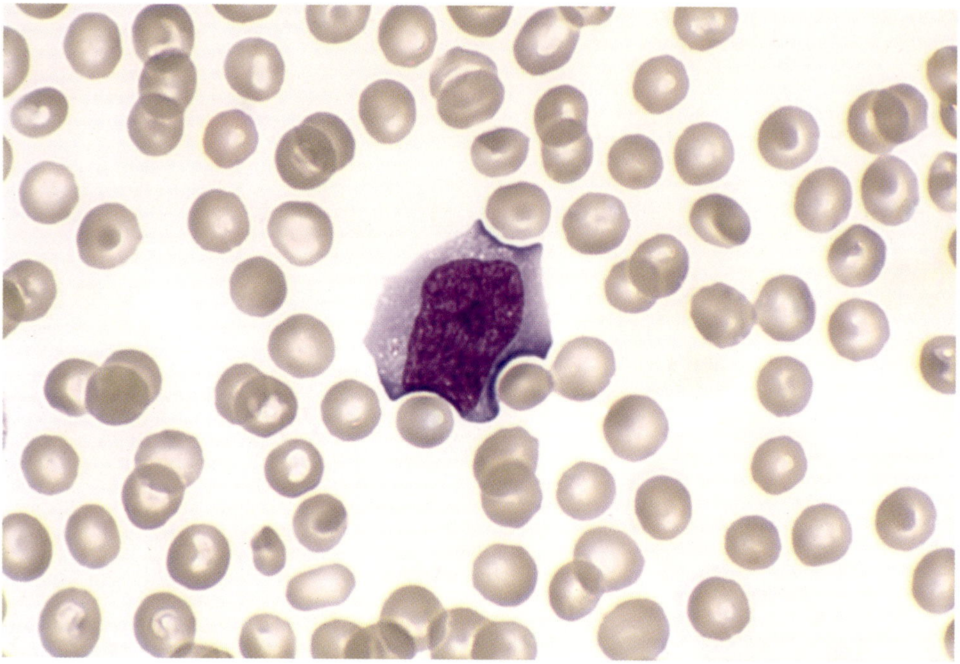

Blood film comments	
Red cell comments	Normal in number and morphology
White blood cell comments	Neutrophilia Reactive lymphocytes
Platelet comments	Occasional large platelet

Question 1. What is the differential diagnosis?

Based on the differential diagnosis, the following tests should be requested

Examination of the blood film

Scan the entire film for the presence of reactive lymphocytes. Be mindful of the fact that the presence of an occasional reactive lymphocyte is suggestive of a prior viral infection giving rise to severe thrombocytopenia in an otherwise healthy child.

The blood film should also be scanned for large or younger platelets, the presence of which suggests that the marrow is trying to compensate for the severe thrombocytopenia.

Bone marrow and trephine

A marrow is performed to ascertain the number of megakaryocytes. In idiopathic thrombocytopenic purpura, megakaryocytes are either normal or increased in number. The low platelet count is secondary to peripheral destruction. Idiopathic thrombocytopenic purpura is an acute self-limiting disease usually resolving over a period of 6 months.

Question 2. Are further tests indicated as part of your final report? If so, which tests?

CASE STUDY 76

Case history
A 2-year-old child presents with empyema.

Analyser data

Parameters	Test Results		Reference Range	
RBC	3.87	$\times 10^{12}$/L	3.86–5.01	$\times 10^{12}$/L
Hb	93	g/L	107–136	g/L
HCT	0.280		0.31–0.38	
MCV	72.4	fL	73–85	fL
MCH	24.0	pg	24.8–29.9	pg
MCHC	332	g/L	310–360	g/L
RDW-SD	35.7	fL	34.8–44.6	fL
RDW-CV	13.6	%	12.3–17.0	%
RETIC CT				
RETIC ABS				
WBC	23.6	$\times 10^9$/L	4.9–12.8	$\times 10^9$/L
Plat	1158	$\times 10^9$/L	214–483	$\times 10^9$/L
ESR	130	mm/h	<10	mm/h

Differential

Parameters	Test Results				Reference Range	
Neutrophil	80.0	%	18.8	$\times 10^9$/L	1.7–6.7	$\times 10^9$/L
Lymphocyte	17.1	%	4.0	$\times 10^9$/L	2.0–6.6	$\times 10^9$/L
Monocyte	2.6	%	0.6	$\times 10^9$/L	0.2–1.0	$\times 10^9$/L
Eosinophil	0.1	%	0.1	$\times 10^9$/L	0.00–0.60	$\times 10^9$/L
Basophil	0.2	%	0.1	$\times 10^9$/L	0.00–0.10	$\times 10^9$/L

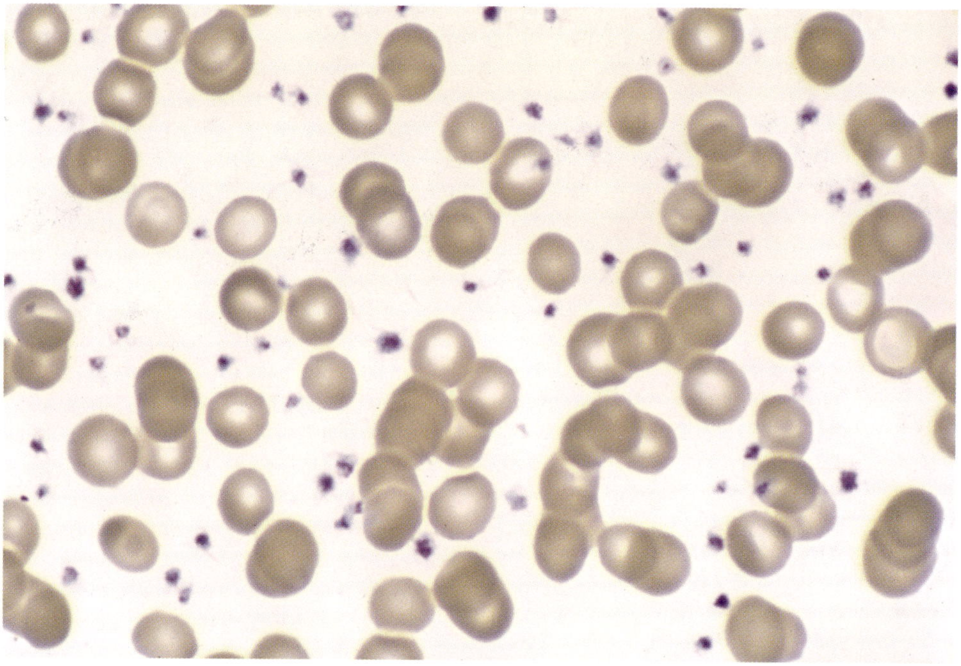

Blood film comments	
Red cell comments	Slight microcytes Slight hypochromasia Marked rouleaux It would be inappropriate to suggest iron studies on a 2-year-old child with the above MCV and MCH.
White blood cell comments	Neutrophilia Slight toxic granulation
Platelet comments	Thrombocytosis Note the platelets are uniform in size; the MPV and PDW are within the reference range.

Question 1. What is the differential diagnosis?

Based on the differential diagnosis, the following tests should be requested
The clinical history, absolute neutrophilia and high ESR are all contributing factors to a diagnosis of reactive thrombocytosis. Note that, unlike the platelets seen in a myeloproliferative neoplasm, the platelets in reactive thrombocytosis are uniform in size. The platelet count usually parallels the severity of the underlying cause.

Question 2. Are further tests indicated as part of your final report? If so, which tests?

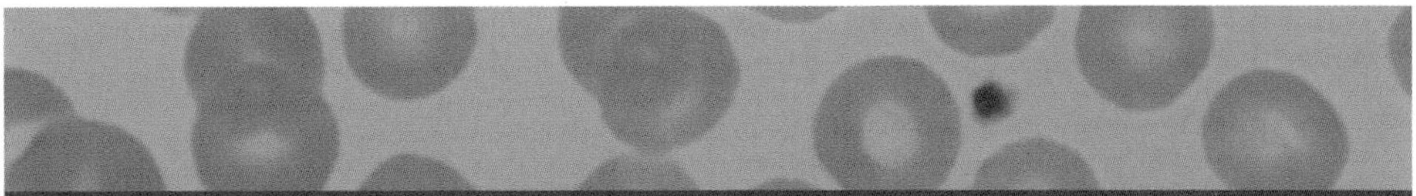

5
Malaria Cases

CASE STUDY 77

Case history

A 23-year-old male returns from New Guinea with fevers and lassitude.

Analyser data				
Parameters	**Test Results**		**Reference Range**	
RBC	4.02	$\times 10^{12}/L$	4.50–6.50	$\times 10^{12}/L$
Hb	113	g/L	130–180	g/L
HCT	0.340		0.40–0.54	
MCV	84.6	fL	80–100	fL
MCH	28.1	pg	26.5–33.0	pg
MCHC	332	g/L	310–360	g/L
RDW-SD	47.7	fL	38.0–48.0	fL
RDW-CV	14.1	%	12.0–14.5	%
RETIC CT				
RETIC ABS				
WBC	3.5	$\times 10^9/L$	3.5–11.0	$\times 10^9/L$
Plat	69	$\times 10^9/L$	150–400	$\times 10^9/L$

Differential						
Parameters	**Test Results**				**Reference Range**	
Neutrophil	62.2	%	2.2	$\times 10^9/L$	1.7–7.0	$\times 10^9/L$
Lymphocyte	28.1	%	1.0	$\times 10^9/L$	1.5–4.0	$\times 10^9/L$
Monocyte	7.4	%	0.3	$\times 10^9/L$	0.1–0.8	$\times 10^9/L$
Eosinophil	2.3	%	0.1	$\times 10^9/L$	0.04–0.44	$\times 10^9/L$
Basophil	0.0	%	0.00	$\times 10^9/L$	0.00–0.20	$\times 10^9/L$

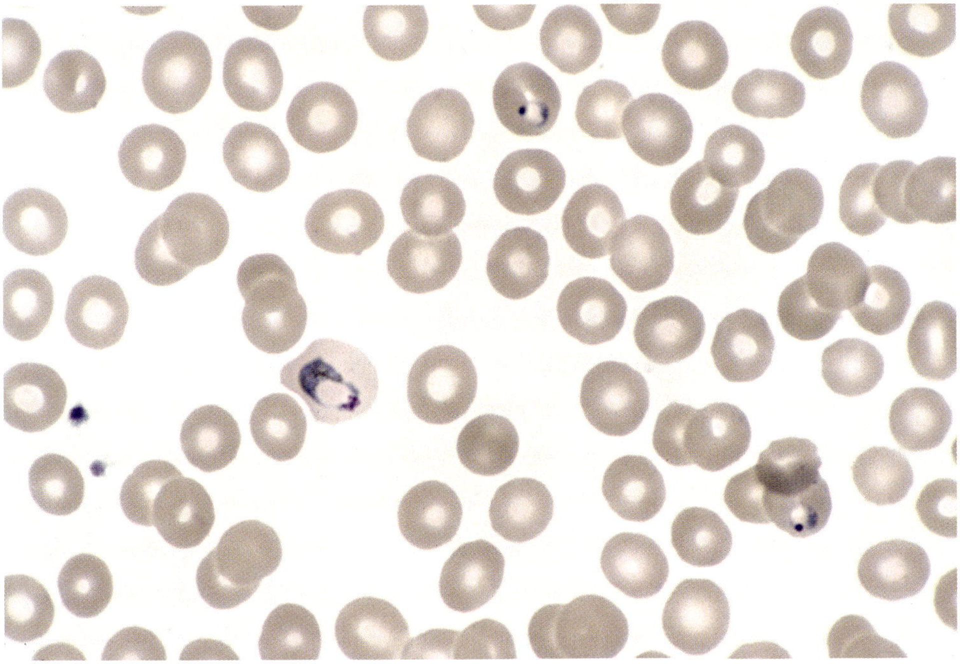

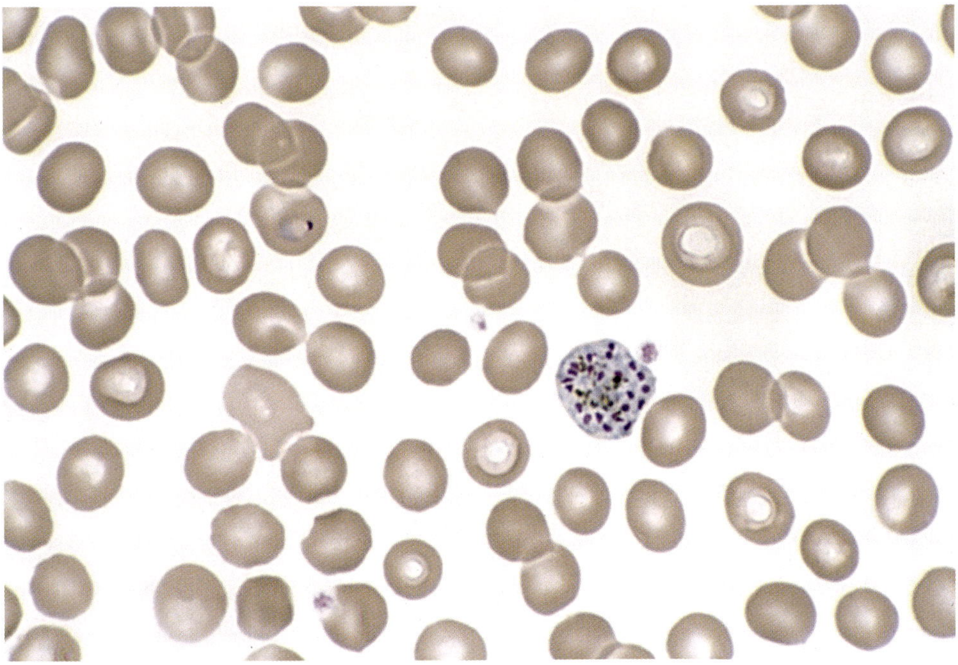

Blood film comments	
Red cell comments	Normal red cell morphology Malarial parasites Early trophozoites and schizonts in enlarged red cells
White blood cell comments	Leucopenia
Platelet comments	Thrombocytopenia

Question 1. What is the differential diagnosis?

Based in the differential diagnosis, the following tests should be requested
ICT screen
An immunochromatographic test (ICT) or rapid diagnostic screening test developed to detect circulating malarial antigens may be performed; however, it must be emphasised that microscopic detection of malarial parasites is the gold standard.
Romanowsky stain with pH 7.2 buffer
At this pH, Schuffner's dots will be visible in both *vivax* and *ovale* malaria, thus their presence will confirm either of the above. The early trophozoites have thickened cytoplasm with a large chromatin dot. This is a case of *Plasmodium vivax*.
Travel history
It is often difficult to differentiate between *vivax* and *ovale* malaria. Travel history can often contribute to a diagnosis.

Question 2. Are further tests indicated as part of your final report? If so, which tests?

CASE STUDY 78

Case history
A 34-year-old female returns from the Solomon Islands with fever and myalgia.

Analyser data				
Parameters	**Test Results**		**Reference Range**	
RBC	2.78	$\times 10^{12}/L$	3.80–5.80	$\times 10^{12}/L$
Hb	80	g/L	115–165	g/L
HCT	0.256		0.37–0.47	
MCV	92.1	fL	80–100	fL
MCH	28.8	pg	26.5–33.0	pg
MCHC	313	g/L	310–360	g/L
RDW-SD	42.6	fL	38.0–48.0	fL
RDW-CV	14.5	%	12.0–14.5	%
RETIC CT				
RETIC ABS				
WBC	3.2	$\times 10^9/L$	3.5–11.0	$\times 10^9/L$
Plat	33	$\times 10^9/L$	150–400	$\times 10^9/L$

Differential						
Parameters	**Test Results**				**Reference Range**	
Neutrophil	73.0	%	2.3	$\times 10^9/L$	1.7–7.0	$\times 10^9/L$
Lymphocyte	22.3	%	0.7	$\times 10^9/L$	1.5–4.0	$\times 10^9/L$
Monocyte	2.8	%	0.1	$\times 10^9/L$	0.1–0.8	$\times 10^9/L$
Eosinophil	1.3	%	0.1	$\times 10^9/L$	0.04–0.44	$\times 10^9/L$
Basophil	0.6	%	0.1	$\times 10^9/L$	0.00–0.20	$\times 10^9/L$

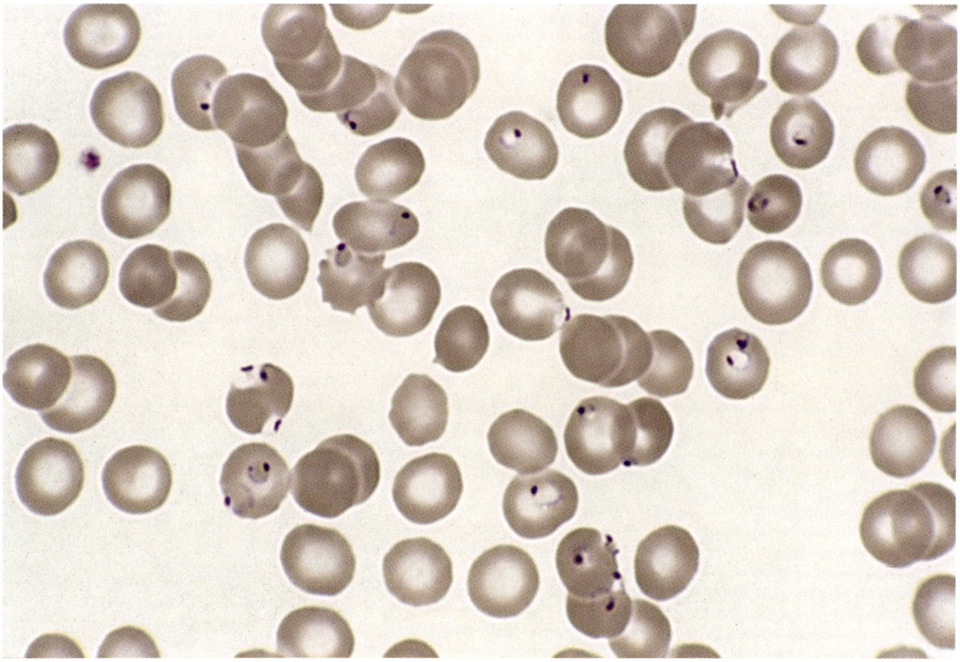

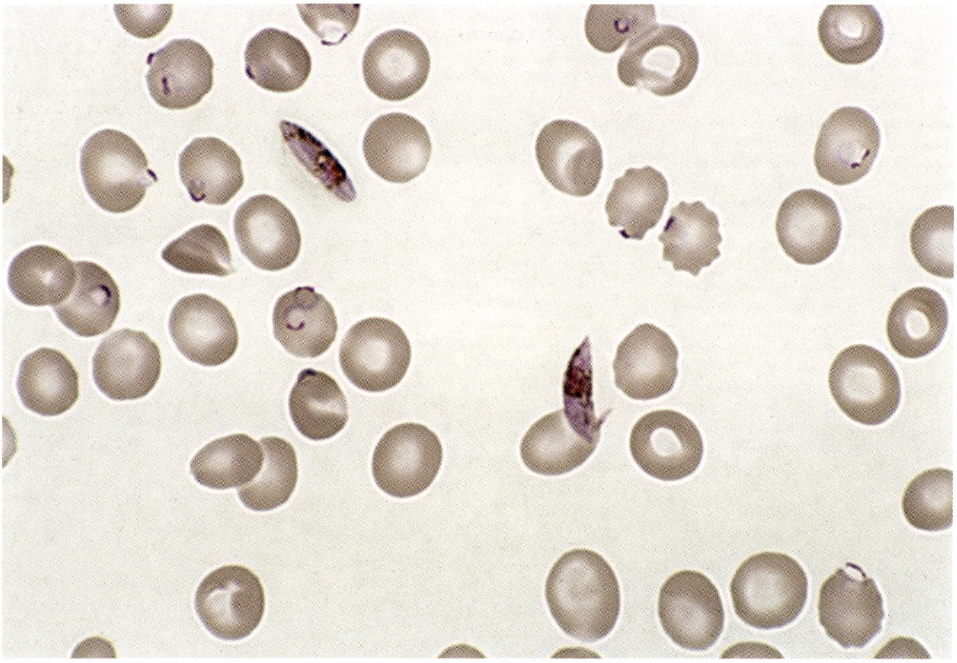

Blood film comments	
Red cell comments	Normal red cell morphology Malarial parasites Early trophozoites and gametocytes in non-enlarged red cells
White blood cell comments	Leucopenia
Platelet comments	Thrombocytopenia

Question 1. What is the differential diagnosis?

Based in the differential diagnosis, the following tests should be requested
ICT screen
An immunochromatographic test (ICT) or rapid diagnostic screening test developed to detect circulating malarial antigens may be performed; however, it must be emphasised that microscopic detection of malarial parasites is the gold standard.
Romanowsky stain with pH 7.2 buffer
At this pH, Schuffner's dots will be visible in both *vivax* and *ovale* malaria and not in *Plasmodium falciparum* malaria. Schuffner's dots are not seen in this case. Morphologically, the early trophozoites are fine and in non-enlarged red cells. Also the gametocytes are crescent-shaped, confirming this to be a case of *Plasmodium falciparum* malaria. This is a case of cerebral *Plasmodium falciparum* malaria.
Travel history
Travel history can often contribute to a diagnosis.

Question 2. Are further tests indicated as part of your final report? If so, which tests?

CASE STUDY 79

Case history

An 18-year-old female returns from Ghana with myalgia and night sweats.

Analyser data				
Parameters	**Test Results**		**Reference Range**	
RBC	3.35	$\times 10^{12}/L$	3.80–5.80	$\times 10^{12}/L$
Hb	94	g/L	115–165	g/L
HCT	0.293		0.37–0.47	
MCV	87.5	fL	80–100	fL
MCH	28.1	pg	26.5–33.0	pg
MCHC	321	g/L	310–360	g/L
RDW-SD	41.2	fL	38.0–48.0	fL
RDW-CV	14.1	%	12.0–14.5	%
RETIC CT				
RETIC ABS				
WBC	2.8	$\times 10^9/L$	3.5–11.0	$\times 10^9/L$
Plat	102	$\times 10^9/L$	150–400	$\times 10^9/L$

Differential						
Parameters	**Test Results**				**Reference Range**	
Neutrophil	96.0	%	2.7	$\times 10^9/L$	1.7–7.0	$\times 10^9/L$
Lymphocyte	3.9	%	0.1	$\times 10^9/L$	1.5–4.0	$\times 10^9/L$
Monocyte	0.4	%	0.1	$\times 10^9/L$	0.1–0.8	$\times 10^9/L$
Eosinophil	0.0	%	0.00	$\times 10^9/L$	0.04–0.44	$\times 10^9/L$
Basophil	0.0	%	0.00	$\times 10^9/L$	0.00–0.20	$\times 10^9/L$

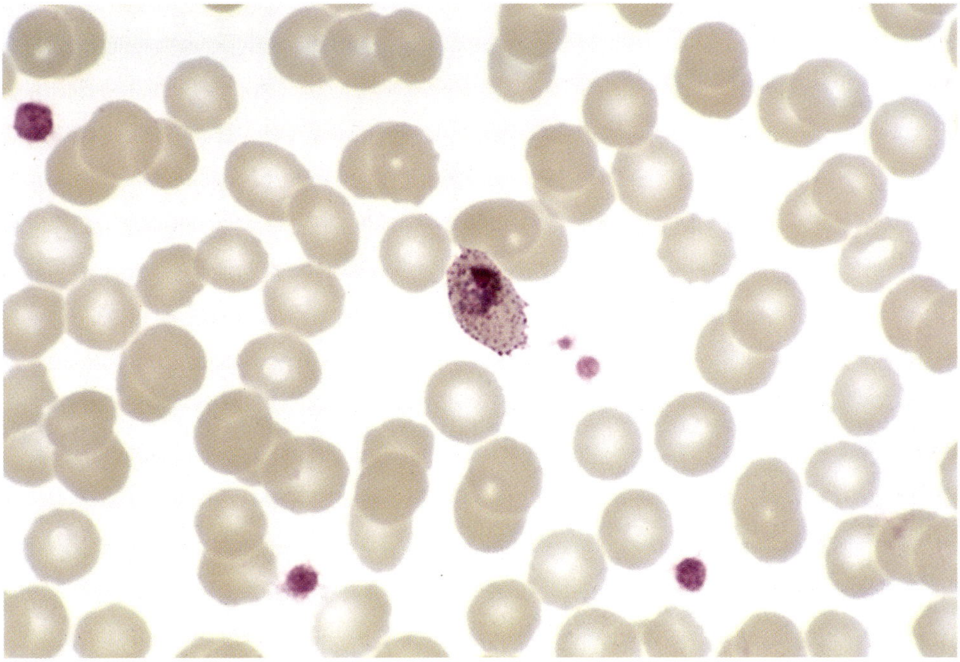

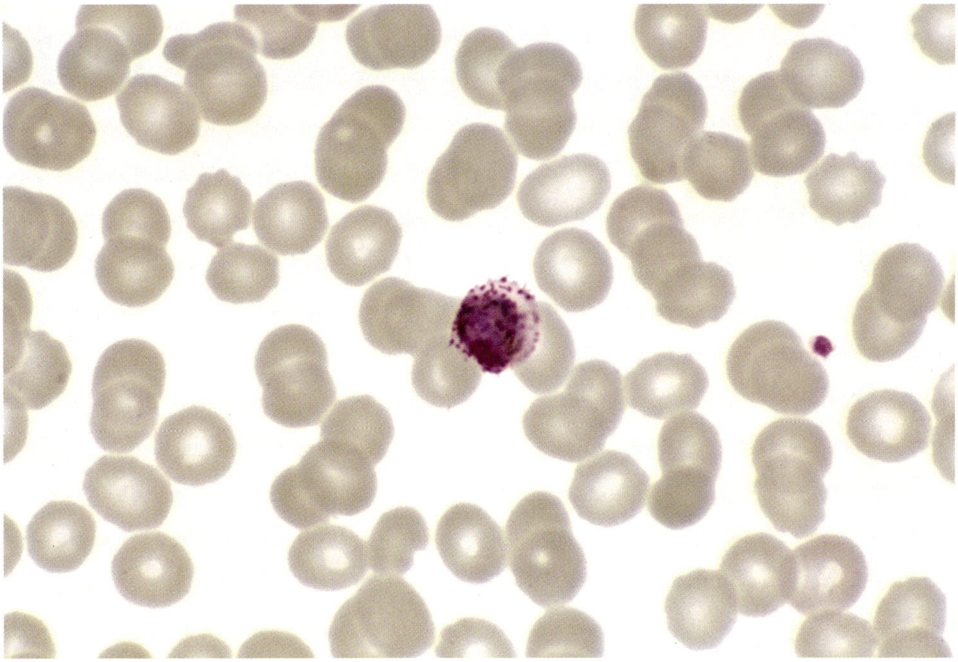

Blood film comments	
Red cell comments	Normal red cell morphology Malarial parasites Late trophozoites and gametocytes in enlarged red cells Schuffner's dots
White blood cell comments	Leucopenia
Platelet comments	Thrombocytopenia

Question 1. What is the differential diagnosis?

Based in the differential diagnosis, the following tests should be requested
ICT screen
An immunochromatographic test (ICT) or rapid diagnostic screening test developed to detect circulating malarial antigens may be performed; however, it must be emphasised that microscopic detection of malarial parasites is the gold standard.
Romanowsky stain with pH 7.2 buffer
At this pH, Schuffner's dots will be visible in both *ovale* and *vivax* malaria thus their presence will confirm either or both *ovale* and *vivax* malaria. Schuffner's dots are present in this case. Morphologically, the late trophozoites and gametocytes of *ovale* tend to be compact within the red cell, taking up about two-thirds of the cell, whereas the late trophozoites and gametocytes of *vivax* tend to fill the entire red cell. In this case, the late trophozoite and gametocyte are compact within the red cell.
Travel history
It is often difficult to differentiate between *ovale* and *vivax* malaria. Travel history can often contribute to a diagnosis.

Question 2. Are further tests indicated as part of your final report? If so, which tests?

CASE STUDY 80

Case history

A 35-year-old male returns from South America where he has been living for two years. He has been having night sweats for a period of 6 months.

Analyser data				
Parameters	**Test Results**		**Reference Range**	
RBC	4.23	$\times 10^{12}/L$	4.50–6.50	$\times 10^{12}/L$
Hb	127	$\times 10^{12}/L$	130–180	$\times 10^{12}/L$
HCT	0.362		0.40–0.54	
MCV	85.6	fL	80–100	fL
MCH	30.0	pg	26.5–33.0	pg
MCHC	350	g/L	310–360	g/L
RDW-SD	47.8	fL	38.0–48.0	fL
RDW-CV	14.1	%	12.0–14.5	%
RETIC CT				
RETIC ABS				
WBC	7.5	$\times 10^9/L$	3.5–11.0	$\times 10^9/L$
Plat	155	$\times 10^9/L$	150–400	$\times 10^9/L$

Differential						
Parameters	**Test Results**				**Reference Range**	
Neutrophil	70.5	%	5.3	$\times 10^9/L$	1.7–7.0	$\times 10^9/L$
Lymphocyte	19.8	%	1.5	$\times 10^9/L$	1.5–4.0	$\times 10^9/L$
Monocyte	7.3	%	0.6	$\times 10^9/L$	0.1–0.8	$\times 10^9/L$
Eosinophil	2.1	%	0.2	$\times 10^9/L$	0.04–0.44	$\times 10^9/L$
Basophil	0.3	%	0.1	$\times 10^9/L$	0.00–0.20	$\times 10^9/L$

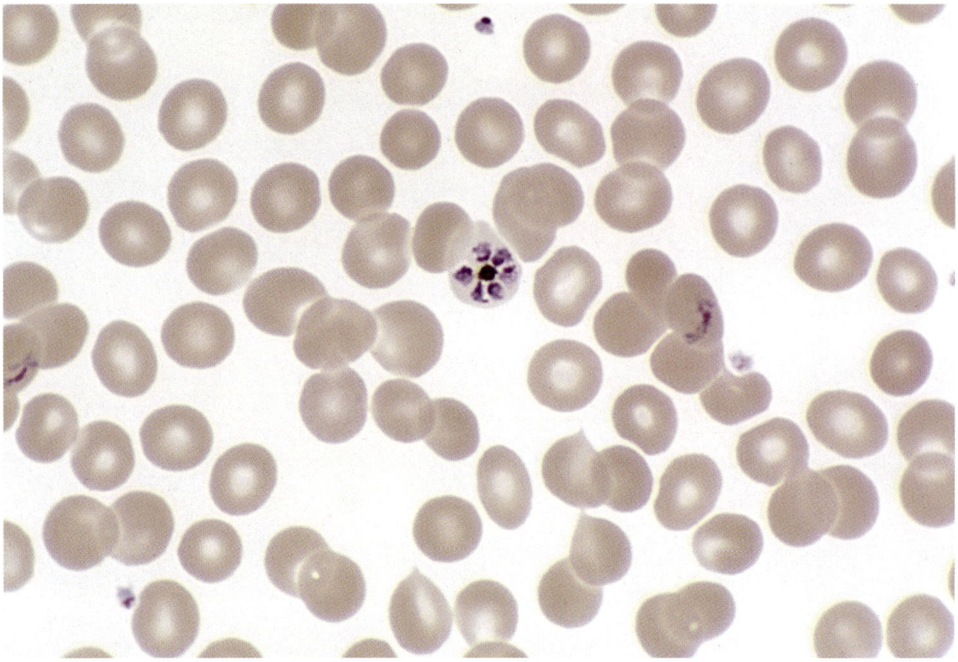

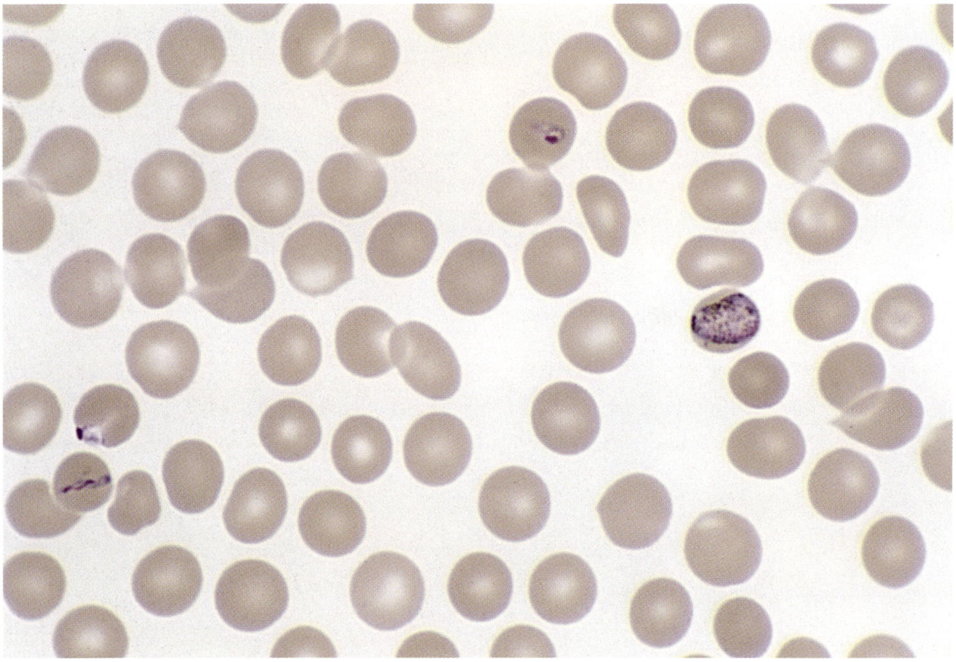

Blood film comments	
Red cell comments	Normal red cell morphology Malarial parasites Early trophozoites, band form trophozoites, schizonts and gametocytes in non-enlarged red cells
White blood cell comments	Normal in number and morphology
Platelets comments	Normal in number and morphology

Question 1. What is the differential diagnosis?

Based in the differential diagnosis, the following tests should be requested
ICT screen An immunochromatographic test (ICT) or rapid diagnostic screening test developed to detect circulating malarial antigens may be performed; however, it must be emphasised that microscopic detection of malarial parasites is the gold standard.
Romanowsky stain with pH 7.2 buffer At this pH, Schuffner's dots will be visible in both *vivax* and *ovale* malaria, thus their presence will confirm either or both *vivax* and *ovale* malaria. There are no Schuffner's dots in this case. The schizont in this case has the classical daisy-head appearance as seen in *Plasmodium malariae*. Band form trophozoites are commonly seen in *Plasmodium malariae*.
Travel history Travel history can often contribute to a diagnosis.

Question 2. Are further tests indicated as part of your final report? If so, which tests?

Answers

2 Red Cell Cases

Case study 1

1. There is no differential diagnosis. Red cells, white cells and platelets are normal in number and morphology.
2. No further tests are indicated.

Actual outcome

Normal adult blood film. This case should be used as a baseline for normality.

Case study 2

1. Iron deficiency anaemia is the most likely diagnosis. The clinical history, together with a microcytic, hypochromic anaemia with elliptocytes, pencil cells and thrombocytosis, are all classical features of chronic blood loss or iron deficiency anaemia.
2. No further tests are indicated.

Actual outcome

Iron deficiency anaemia

Case study 3

1. The blood film image in this case is dimorphic. There are two populations of red cells, namely microcytic hypochromic and normocytic normochromic; hence the raised RDW. There is no differential diagnosis.
2. No further tests are indicated.

Actual outcome

Dimorphic blood film (partially treated iron deficiency anaemia)

Case study 4

1. Megaloblastic anaemia (B_{12} and/or folic acid deficiency)
2. Test for intrinsic factor blocking antibody to diagnose pernicious anaemia.

Actual outcome

Megaloblastic anaemia (vitamin B_{12} deficiency)

Case study 5

1. Megaloblastic anaemia (B_{12} and/or folic acid deficiency)
2. No further tests are indicated.

Actual outcome

Nutritional anaemia (B_{12} and folic acid deficiency)

Case study 6

1. Liver disease
2. No further tests are indicated.

Actual outcome

Liver disease (alcoholic)

Case study 7

1. The blood film, together with the marked thrombocytopenia, is consistent with spur cell anaemia.
2. No further tests are indicated.

Actual outcome

Spur cell anaemia. Note that spur cell anaemia is characterised by a marked thrombocytopenia due to the lack of thrombopoietin being produced by a damaged liver. The liver enzymes are also reduced secondary to the damaged liver. Spur cell anaemia is consistent with fulminant liver failure.

Case study 8

1. Paroxysmal nocturnal haemoglobinuria; aplastic anaemia
2. No further tests are indicated.

Actual outcome

Paroxysmal nocturnal haemoglobinuria

Case study 9

1. Hereditary spherocytosis; autoimmune haemolytic anaemia
2. Family studies

Actual outcome

Hereditary spherocytosis

Case study 10

1. Autoimmune haemolytic anaemia
2. No further tests are indicated.

Actual outcome

Autoimmune haemolytic anaemia

Case study 11

1. ABO haemolytic disease of the newborn; hereditary spherocytosis
2. No further tests are indicated.

Actual outcome

ABO haemolytic disease of the newborn

Case study 12

1. Rh haemolytic disease of the newborn
2. No further tests are indicated.

Actual outcome

Rh haemolytic disease of the newborn

Case study 13

1. Hereditary pyropoikilocytosis (HPP)
2. Family studies

Actual outcome

Hereditary pyropoikilocytosis

Case study 14

1. *Clostridium perfringens* sepsis
2. No further tests are indicated. Refer to microbiology results at a later date.

Actual outcome

Clostridium perfringens sepsis

Case study 15

1. Microangiopathic haemolytic anaemia (haemolytic uraemic syndrome (HUS) or thrombotic thrombocytopenic purpura (TTP))
2. No further tests are indicated.

Actual outcome

Microangiopathic haemolytic anaemia; haemolytic uraemic syndrome (HUS). Clinically, a diagnosis of TTP would have been made if this child had demonstrated neurological signs such as going in and out of consciousness. The red cell changes in HUS and TTP are indistinguishable.

Case study 16

1. Microangiopathic haemolytic anaemia (thrombotic thrombocytopenic purpura (TTP) or haemolytic uraemic syndrome (HUS))
2. No further tests are indicated.

Actual outcome

Microangiopathic haemolytic anaemia; thrombotic thrombocytopenic purpura. Clinically, this child has neurological signs and hence a diagnosis of TTP was made. The red cell changes in HUS and TTP are indistinguishable.

Case study 17

1. Microangiopathic haemolytic anaemia secondary to heart valve haemolysis
2. No further tests are indicated.

Actual outcome

Microangiopathic haemolytic anaemia; heart valve haemolysis. Note that the platelet count is invariably normal in heart valve haemolysis.

Case study 18

1. Microangiopathic haemolytic anaemia secondary to HELLP syndrome
2. No further tests are indicated.

Actual outcome

Microangiopathic haemolytic anaemia secondary to HELLP syndrome

Case study 19

1. Oxidant haemolysis; G6PD deficiency
2. A Heinz body preparation (methyl violet/cresyl blue) may be performed for the detection of Heinz bodies. The Heinz body preparation shown in this case study does not come from the above neonate. It comes from a patient who has had a splenectomy and who was taking Dapsone, an oxidant drug for idiopathic thrombocytopenic purpura (ITP); hence the number of intact cells containing Heinz bodies.

Actual outcome

Oxidant haemolysis

Case study 20

1. Iron deficiency, thalassaemia, or a combination of both
2. Iron studies should always be performed in conjunction with the Hb EPG. The iron studies in this case study were normal. Family studies.

Actual outcome

Alpha thalassaemia trait

Case study 21

1. Iron deficiency anaemia; thalassaemia trait
2. Iron studies should always be performed in conjunction with the Hb EPG. The iron studies in this case study were normal. Family studies.

Actual outcome

Beta thalassaemia trait

Case study 22

1. Iron deficiency anaemia; thalassaemia trait
2. Iron studies should always be performed in conjunction with the Hb EPG. The iron studies in this case study were normal. Family studies.

Actual outcome

Haemoglobin H disease

Case study 23

1. Thalassaemia trait; haemoglobin Hb Constant Spring
2. Family studies

Actual outcome

Haemoglobin Hb Constant Spring

Case study 24

1. Beta thalassaemia intermedia; thalassaemia major
2. Family studies

Actual outcome

Beta thalassaemia intermedia. The iron studies are consistent with multiple red cell transfusions.

Case study 25

1. Beta thalassaemia major; beta thalassaemia intermedia
2. Family studies

Actual outcome

Beta thalassaemia major. The iron studies are consistent with multiple red cell transfusions.

Case study 26

1. Thalassaemia trait; iron deficiency anaemia
2. Family studies

Actual outcome

Haemoglobin E trait

Case study 27

1. HbEE disease. The low MCV and marked number of target cells are suggestive of HbEE.
2. Family studies

Actual outcome

Haemoglobin EE disease

Case study 28

1. Haemoglobin SS disease
2. Family studies

Actual outcome

Haemoglobin SS disease. The iron studies are consistent with multiple red cell transfusions.
Note that the majority of cases will also show features of auto splenectomy. When the red cells containing HbS enter the fine capillaries of the body, they become deoxygenated, change shape, and block off those fine capillaries. This process leads to splenic infarcts or cell deaths throughout the spleen. Hence Howell Jolly bodies, Pappenheimer bodies and the characteristic red cell changes seen in hyposplenism will also be seen in HbSS.

Case study 29

1. Haemoglobin CC disease; iron deficiency anaemia
2. Family studies

Actual outcome

Haemoglobin CC disease

Case study 30

1. There is no differential diagnosis. The image is diagnostic.
2. No further tests are indicated.

Actual outcome

Third degree burns to 75% of the body

Case study 31

1. Hereditary elliptocytosis
2. As the image is diagnostic of hereditary elliptocytosis one would not pursue further testing; however, flow cytometry using eosin 5 maleimide could be performed to detect the level of spectrin and protein 4.1 within the red cell membrane. Family studies.

Actual outcome

Hereditary elliptocytosis

Case study 32

1. Southeast Asian ovalocytosis
2. As the image is diagnostic of Southeast Asian ovalocytosis one would not pursue further testing; however, flow cytometry using eosin 5 maleimide could be performed to detect the level of ankyrin and protein 3 mobility within the red cell membrane. Family studies.

Actual outcome

Southeast Asian ovalocytosis

Case study 33

1. Hereditary stomatocytosis; splenectomy/hyposplenism
2. Flow cytometry using eosin 5 maleimide should be performed to detect the level of protein 7.2b or stomatin within the red cell membrane. Family studies. This patient came to the casualty department with a history of hereditary stomatocytosis for which he was splenectomised at the age of 8 years.

Actual outcome

Hereditary stomatocytosis; splenectomy

Case study 34

1. Abetalipoproteinaemia; McLeod phenotype
2. No further tests are indicated.

Actual outcome

Abetalipoproteinaemia

Case study 35

1. Normochromic, normocytic anaemia
2. No further tests are indicated.

Actual outcome

Chronic renal failure

Case study 36

1. Acute renal failure
2. No further tests are indicated.

Actual outcome

Acute renal failure

Case study 37

1. Splenectomy; hyposplenism
2. No further tests are indicated.

Actual outcome

Post splenectomy (secondary to trauma)

3 White Cell Cases

Case study 38

1. A myeloproliferative neoplasm such as chronic myelogenous leukaemia, *BCR-ABL 1* positive. The peripheral blood film in the chronic phase of chronic myelogenous leukaemia, *BCR-ABL 1* positive shows approximately 50% neutrophils while the less mature myeloid cells are present in diminishing frequency with less than 2% blasts and a basophilia.
2. No further tests are indicated.

Actual outcome

Myeloproliferative neoplasm. Chronic myelogenous leukaemia, *BCR-ABL 1* positive.

Case study 39

1. A myeloproliferative neoplasm such as polycythaemia vera
2. Iron studies may be indicated. (Therapeutic venesection and/or chronic gastrointestinal bleeding can result in iron deficiency.)

Actual outcome

Polycythaemia vera (pre-polycythaemic phase/overt polycythaemia)

Case study 40

1. A myeloproliferative neoplasm such as primary myelofibrosis. A leucoerythroblastic blood picture with teardrop poikilocytes is characteristic of primary myelofibrosis and/or metastatic carcinoma.
2. No further tests are indicated.

Actual outcome

Primary myelofibrosis (fibrotic stage)

Case study 41

1. Essential thrombocythaemia (ET). (Large and giant platelets are characteristic of ET while the platelets in reactive thrombocytosis are uniform in size.)
2. No further tests are indicated although iron studies may be performed.

Actual outcome

Essential thrombocythaemia

Case study 42

1. A myelodysplastic/myeloproliferative neoplasm such as juvenile myelomonocytic leukaemia
2. No further tests are indicated.

Actual outcome

Juvenile myelomonocytic leukaemia (JMML)
JMML is characterised by:

- monocytosis
- raised HbF
- Philadelphia chromosome negative.

Case study 43

1. A myelodysplastic/myeloproliferative neoplasm such as chronic myelomonocytic leukaemia
2. No further tests are indicated.

Actual outcome

Chronic myelomonocytic leukaemia (CMML-1)

Case study 44

1. Myelodysplastic syndrome/neoplasm
2. No further tests are indicated.

Actual outcome

Myelodysplastic syndrome. Refractory cytopenia with unilineage dysplasia (refractory anaemia).

Case study 45

1. Myelodysplastic syndrome/neoplasm
2. No further tests are indicated.

Actual outcome

Myelodysplastic syndrome. Refractory cytopenia with multilineage dysplasia.

Case study 46

1. Viral infection
2. No further tests are indicated.

Actual outcome

Infectious mononucleosis (Epstein Barr virus infection)

Case study 47

1. Viral infection; varicella
2. No further tests are indicated.

Actual outcome

Varicella zoster-chicken pox

Case study 48

1. Malaria; infectious mononucleosis; viral infection such as dengue fever
2. No further tests are indicated.

Actual outcome

Dengue fever

Case study 49

1. *Bordetella pertussis* infection; acute infectious lymphocytosis of childhood
2. No further tests are indicated.

Actual outcome

Bordetella pertussis (whooping cough)

Case study 50

1. B-cell chronic lymphocytic leukaemia/small lymphocytic lymphoma
2. No further tests are indicated. The immunophenotyping confirms B-chronic lymphocytic leukaemia/small lymphocytic lymphoma.

Actual outcome

B-chronic lymphocytic leukaemia/small lymphocytic lymphoma

Case study 51

1. B-cell prolymphocytic leukaemia
2. No further tests are indicated. The immunophenotyping confirms B-cell prolymphocytic leukaemia.

Actual outcome

B-cell prolymphocytic leukaemia

Case study 52

1. Splenic B-cell marginal zone lymphoma; hairy cell leukaemia
2. No further tests are indicated. The immunophenotyping confirms splenic B-cell marginal zone lymphoma.

Actual outcome

Splenic B-cell marginal zone lymphoma

Case study 53

1. Hairy cell leukaemia (variant); splenic B-cell marginal zone lymphoma
2. No further tests are indicated. The immunophenotyping confirms the variant form of hairy cell leukaemia.

Actual outcome

Hairy cell leukaemia (variant form)

Case study 54

1. Non-Hodgkin lymphoma
2. No further tests are indicated. The immunophenotyping confirms non-Hodgkin lymphoma (follicular lymphoma).

Actual outcome

Non-Hodgkin lymphoma (follicular lymphoma)

Case study 55

1. Non-Hodgkin lymphoma
2. No further tests are indicated. The immunophenotyping confirms non-Hodgkin lymphoma (mantle cell lymphoma).

Actual outcome

Non-Hodgkin lymphoma (mantle cell lymphoma)

Case study 56

1. A leucoerythroblastic blood film suggests bone marrow infiltration, thus a bone marrow needs to be performed in this case. There is no differential diagnosis at this stage.
2. Immunophenotyping confirms Burkitt cell leukaemia. Further tests are indicated:
   (a) Screen for the Epstein Barr virus antibody (sporadic Burkitt lymphoma).
   (b) Screen for HTLV 1+2 antibody (immunodeficiency associated Burkitt lymphoma).

Actual outcome

Burkitt cell leukaemia

Case study 57

1. Plasma cell myeloma; plasmacytoma
2. Immunophenotyping confirms plasma cell myeloma. Serum proteins and Bence Jones protein in the urine are indicated.

Actual outcome

Plasma cell myeloma

Case study 58

1. Lymphoblastic leukaemia/lymphoma, not otherwise specified
2. No further tests are indicated. Immunophenotyping confirms B lymphoblastic leukaemia (common ALL).

Actual outcome

B lymphoblastic leukaemia/lymphoma, not otherwise specified

Case study 59

1. Lymphoblastic leukaemia/lymphoma, not otherwise specified. Note that T lymphoblastic leukaemia/lymphoma classically presents with a mediastinal mass with a markedly increased white cell count.
2. No further tests are indicated. The immunophenotyping confirms T lymphoblastic leukaemia.

Actual outcome

T lymphoblastic leukaemia/lymphoma, not otherwise specified

Case study 60

1. Septicaemia
2. In view of the marked thrombocytopenia, coagulation studies including D-DIM LIA and fibrinogen should be performed. The thrombocytopenia could be due to disseminated intravascular coagulation (DIC) and/or septicaemia. In this case the coagulation studies were normal. The thrombocytopenia is secondary to septicaemia.

Actual outcome

Septicaemia

Case study 61

1. Septicaemia; cytokine/G-CSF therapy
2. No further tests are indicated.

Actual outcome

Cytokine/G-CSF therapy (child receiving chemotherapy for neuroblastoma)

Case study 62

1. Septicaemia; Kawasaki disease
2. No further tests are indicated.

Actual outcome

Kawasaki disease

Case study 63

1. Acute myeloid leukaemia with recurrent genetic abnormalities; acute promyelocytic leukaemia with t(15;17)(q22;q12) *PML-RARA*
2. Coagulation studies *must* be performed as acute promyelocytic leukaemia is associated with a coagulopathy, namely disseminated intravascular coagulation or DIC.

Actual outcome

Acute promyelocytic leukaemia with t(15;17)(q22;q12) *PML-RARA*.

Case study 64

1. Acute myeloid leukaemia
2. No further tests are indicated. Immunophenotyping confirms acute myeloid leukaemia.

Actual outcome

Acute myeloid leukaemia, not otherwise specified: acute myeloid leukaemia with minimal differentiation

Case study 65

1. Acute myeloid leukaemia
2. No further tests are indicated. Immunophenotyping confirms acute myeloid leukaemia.

Actual outcome

Acute myeloid leukaemia, not otherwise specified: acute myeloid leukaemia without maturation

Case study 66

1. Acute myeloid leukaemia
2. No further tests are indicated. Immunophenotyping confirms acute myeloid leukaemia.

Actual outcome

Acute myeloid leukaemia, not otherwise specified: acute myeloid leukaemia with maturation

Case study 67

1. Acute myeloid leukaemia
2. No further tests are indicated. Immunophenotyping confirms acute myelomonocytic leukaemia.

Actual outcome

Acute myeloid leukaemia, not otherwise specified: acute myelomonocytic leukaemia

Case study 68

1. Acute myeloid leukaemia
2. No further tests are indicated. Immunophenotyping confirms acute monoblastic leukaemia.

Actual outcome

Acute myeloid leukaemia, not otherwise specified: acute monoblastic and monocytic leukaemia

Case study 69

1. Acute myeloid leukaemia
2. No further tests are indicated. Immunophenotyping confirms acute erythroleukaemia (erythroid/myeloid).

Actual outcome

Acute myeloid leukaemia, not otherwise specified: acute erythroleukaemia (erythroid/myeloid)

Case study 70

1. Acute myeloid leukaemia
2. No further tests are indicated. Immunophenotyping confirms acute megakaryoblastic leukaemia.

Actual outcome
Acute myeloid leukaemia, not otherwise specified: acute megakaryoblastic leukaemia

Case study 71

1. Transient abnormal myelopoiesis (TAM); congenital leukaemia
2. No further tests are indicated. Immunophenotyping confirms myeloid leukaemia with megakaryocytic markers, namely CD41 and CD61. The white cell count returned to normal and the blasts disappeared, confirming this to be a case of TAM.

Actual outcome
TAM

4 Platelet Cases

Case study 72

1. May-Hegglin anomaly; Bernard-Soulier syndrome
2. No further tests are indicated.

Actual outcome
May-Hegglin anomaly

Case study 73

1. Bernard-Soulier syndrome; May-Hegglin anomaly
2. No further tests are indicated.

Actual outcome
Bernard-Soulier syndrome

Case study 74

1. Suggestive of Wiskott-Aldrich syndrome
2. Immunoglobulin levels; genetic testing

Actual outcome
Wiskott-Aldrich syndrome

Case study 75

1. Idiopathic thrombocytopenic purpura; acute leukaemia
2. No further tests are indicated.

Actual outcome
Idiopathic thrombocytopenic purpura

Case study 76

1. Reactive thrombocytosis
2. No further tests are indicated.

Actual outcome

Reactive thrombocytosis

5 Malaria Cases

Case study 77

1. *Plasmodium vivax* malaria; *Plasmodium ovale* malaria
2. No further tests are indicated.

Actual outcome

Plasmodium vivax malaria. The images include early trophozoites and a schizont (pH 6.8).

Case study 78

1. *Plasmodium falciparum* malaria
2. No further tests are indicated.

Actual outcome

Plasmodium falciparum malaria. The images include early trophozoites and gametocytes (pH 6.8).

Case study 79

1. *Plasmodium ovale*; *Plasmodium vivax*
2. No further tests are indicated.

Actual outcome

Plasmodium ovale malaria. The images include a late trophozoite and gametocyte showing Schuffner's dots (pH 7.2).

Case study 80

1. *Plasmodium malariae*
2. No further tests are indicated.

Actual outcome

Plasmodium malariae malaria. The images include early trophozoites, band form trophozoites, a schizont, and a gametocyte (pH 6.8).